Study Guide

Understanding Nutrition

THIRTEENTH EDITION

Ellie Whitney

Sharon Rady Rolfes

Prepared by

Lori W. Turner
University of Alabama

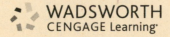

WADSWORTH
CENGAGE Learning·

Australia • Brazil • Japan • Korea • Mexico • Singapore • Spain • United Kingdom • United States

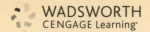
ISBN-13: 978-1-133-60443-3
ISBN-10: 1-133-60443-9

Wadsworth
20 Davis Drive
Belmont, CA 94002-3098
USA

Cengage Learning is a leading provider of customized learning solutions with office locations around the globe, including Singapore, the United Kingdom, Australia, Mexico, Brazil, and Japan. Locate your local office at:
www.cengage.com/global

Cengage Learning products are represented in Canada by Nelson Education, Ltd.

To learn more about Wadsworth, visit
www.cengage.com/wadsworth

Purchase any of our products at your local college store or at our preferred online store
www.cengagebrain.com

Printed in the United States of America
1 2 3 4 5 6 7 16 15 14 13 12

❧ Table of Contents ❧

❧ What's in This Study Guide? ❧

Thank you for purchasing the Study Guide for *Understanding Nutrition*, 13th edition! The exercises in this workbook are designed to help you prepare for examinations by reviewing key concepts and testing your recall of information presented in each textbook chapter. Answers for all questions are provided in an answer key at the end of each Study Guide section. The features of this Study Guide include:

- **Chapter Outlines** – Scan the outline to quickly review the topics covered within the chapter

- **Summing Up** – Fill in the blanks to complete the chapter summary

- **Chapter Study Questions** – Answer these discussion questions to practice explaining important processes and concepts in your own words

- **Key Terms Practice** – Review key terms and definitions from the chapter by completing a crossword puzzle and matching exercise

- **Sample Test Questions** – Take this multiple-choice practice test to see how much you remember

- **Short Answer Questions** – Check your memory with these classifying and listing exercises

- **Problem Solving** – Practice application of chapter concepts through nutrition calculations and other word problems

- **Figure Identification** – Label anatomical diagrams and chemical structures

❦ Chapter 1 ~ An Overview of Nutrition ❧

Chapter Outline

I. Food Choices
  A. Preference
  B. Habit
  C. Ethnic Heritage and Regional Cuisines
  D. Social Interactions
  E. Availability, Convenience, and Economy
  F. Positive and Negative Associations
  G. Emotions
  H. Values
  I. Body Weight and Image
  J. Nutrition and Health Benefits

II. The Nutrients
  A. Nutrients in Foods and in the Body
    1. Nutrient Composition of Foods
    2. Nutrient Composition of the Body
    3. Chemical Composition of Nutrients
    4. Essential Nutrients
  B. The Energy-Yielding Nutrients: Carbohydrate, Fat, and Protein
    1. Energy Measured in kCalories
    2. Energy from Foods
    3. Energy in the Body
    4. Other Roles of Energy-Yielding Nutrients
  C. The Vitamins
  D. The Minerals
  E. Water

III. The Science of Nutrition
  A. Conducting Research
    1. Controls
    2. Sample Size
    3. Placebos
    4. Double Blind
  B. Analyzing Research Findings
    1. Correlations and Causes
    2. Cautious Conclusions
  C. Publishing Research

IV. Dietary Reference Intakes
  A. Establishing Nutrient Recommendations
    1. Estimated Average Requirements (EAR)
    2. Recommended Dietary Allowances (RDA)
    3. Adequate Intakes (AI)
    4. Tolerable Upper Intake Levels (UL)
  B. Establishing Energy Recommendations
    1. Estimated Energy Requirement (EER)
    2. Acceptable Macronutrient Distribution Ranges (AMDR)
  C. Using Nutrient Recommendations
  D. Comparing Nutrient Recommendations

V. Nutrition Assessment
  A. Nutrition Assessment of Individuals
    1. Historical Information
    2. Anthropometric Measurements
    3. Physical Examinations
    4. Laboratory Tests
    5. Iron, for Example
  B. Nutrition Assessment of Populations
    1. National Nutrition Surveys
    2. National Health Goals
    3. National Trends

VI. Diet and Health
  A. Chronic Diseases
  B. Risk Factors for Chronic Diseases
    1. Risk Factors Persist
    2. Risk Factors Cluster
    3. Risk Factors in Perspective
    4. Health Behaviors in the United States

VII. Nutrition Information and Misinformation
  A. Nutrition on the Internet
  B. Nutrition in the News
  C. Identifying Nutrition Experts
    1. Physicians and Other Health-Care Professionals
    2. Registered Dietitian (RD)
    3. Dietetic Technician, Registered (DTR)
    4. Other Dietary Employees
  D. Identifying Fake Credentials
  E. Red Flags of Nutrition Quackery

Summing Up

A person selects foods for a variety of 1. _Reasons_. Whatever those reasons may be, food choices influence 2._____. Individual food selections neither make nor break a diet's

3._____, but the balance of foods selected over time can make an 4._____

difference to health. For this reason, people are wise to think "nutrition" when making their 5._____ choices.

Foods provide 6._____—substances that support the growth, 7._____, and repair of the body's tissues. The six classes of nutrients include: 8._____, lipids (fats), proteins, vitamins, 9._____, and water. Foods rich in the 10._____-_____ nutrients (carbohydrate, fat, and protein) provide the major 11._____ for building the body's tissues and yield 12._____ for the body's use or storage. Energy is measured in 13._____—a measure of heat energy. Vitamins, minerals, and 14._____ do not yield energy; instead they facilitate a variety of activities in the body.

Scientists learn about nutrition by conducting 15._____ that follow the protocol of scientific research. In designing their studies, researchers randomly assign control and 16._____ groups, seek 17._____ sample sizes, provide 18._____, and remain blind to treatments. Their findings must be reviewed and 19._____ by other scientists before being accepted as valid.

The Dietary Reference Intakes (DRI) are a set of nutrient intake values that can be used to plan and 20._____ diets for healthy people. The Estimated Average Requirement (EAR) defines the amount of a nutrient that supports a specific function in the body for 21._____ of the population. The Recommended Dietary Allowance (RDA) is based on the Estimated Average Requirement and establishes a goal for dietary intake that will meet the needs of almost all 22._____ people. An Adequate Intake (AI) serves a similar purpose when an 23._____ cannot be determined. The Estimated Energy Requirement (EER) defines the 24._____ amount of energy intake needed to maintain energy balance, and the Acceptable Macronutrient Distribution Ranges (AMDR) define the 25._____ contributed by carbohydrate, fat, and protein to a healthy diet. The Tolerable Upper Intake Level (UL) establishes the 26._____ amount that appears safe for regular consumption.

People become 27._____ when they get too little or too much energy or nutrients. Deficiencies, excesses, and imbalances of nutrients lead to 28._____ diseases. To detect malnutrition in individuals, health-care professionals use a combination of four nutrition 29._____ methods. Reviewing 30._____ information on diet and health may suggest a possible nutrition problem. Laboratory tests may detect a possible nutrition problem in its 31._____ stages, whereas 32._____ measurements and physical examinations pick up on the problem only after it causes symptoms. National surveys use similar assessment methods to measure people's food consumption and to evaluate the nutrition status of 33._____.

Within the range set by 34._____, a person's choice of diet influences long-term health. Diet has no influence on some diseases but is linked 35._____ to others. Personal life 36._____, such as engaging in physical activity and using tobacco or alcohol, also affect health for the better or worse.

Chapter Study Questions

1. List the various factors that influence personal food choices.

2. What is the number one reason most people choose certain foods? Discuss how people can learn to select foods for nutrition and health benefits.

3. What is a nutrient? Name the six classes of nutrients found in foods. What is an essential nutrient?

4. Which nutrients are inorganic and which are organic? Discuss the significance of that distinction.

5. Which nutrients yield energy and how much energy do they yield per gram? How is energy measured?

6. Describe some roles of energy-yielding nutrients other than providing energy.

7. Describe how alcohol resembles nutrients. Why is alcohol not considered a nutrient?

8. What is the science of nutrition? Define nutritional genomics.

4

9. Describe the scientific method.

10. Name the types of research studies and methods used in acquiring nutrition information.

11. Explain how association between variables might be correlational but not causal. Define positive and negative correlations.

12. What are the DRI? Who develops the DRI? To whom do they apply? How are they used?

13. Identify the four categories of DRI and indicate how they are related.

14. What judgment factors are involved in setting the energy and nutrient intake recommendations?

15. What happens when people either get too little or too much energy or nutrients? Define malnutrition, undernutrition, and overnutrition. List the four methods used to detect energy and nutrient deficiencies and excesses.

16. What methods are used in nutrition surveys? What kinds of information can these surveys provide?

17. Describe risk factors and their relationships to disease.

18. Discuss what researchers know about risk factors in terms of the way they persist and cluster. How has this knowledge affected people's behavior in the United States?

Key Terms Practice

To complete the crossword puzzle, identify the key term that best matches each definition.

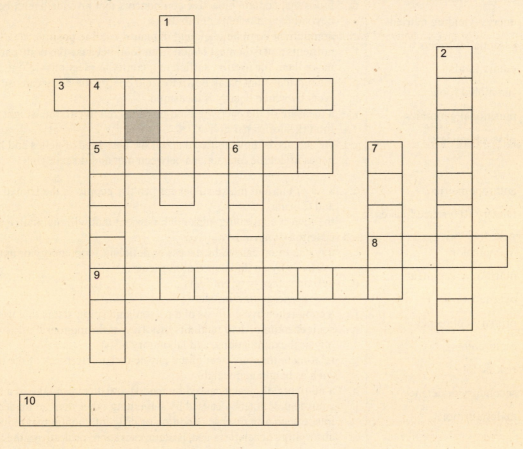

Across:
3. Inorganic elements, some of which are essential nutrients required in small amounts by the body for health.
5. In chemistry, a substance or molecule containing carbon-carbon bonds or carbon-hydrogen bonds.
8. The foods and beverages a person eats and drinks.
9. Chemical substances obtained from food and used in the body to provide energy, structural materials, and regulating agents to support growth, maintenance, and repair of the body's tissues.
10. Organic, essential nutrients required in small amounts by the body for health.

Down:
1. The capacity to do work. The chemical form in the body can be converted to mechanical, electrical, or heat forms.
2. The amount of a nutrient below which almost all healthy people can be expected, over time, to experience deficiency symptoms.
4. Not containing carbon or pertaining to living things.
6. The science of the nutrients in foods and their actions within the body. A broader definition includes the study of human behaviors related to food and eating.

6

7. Products derived from plants or animals that can be taken into the body to yield energy and nutrients for the maintenance of life and the growth and repair of tissues.

Match the key terms with their definitions.

11. _____ calories

12. _____ chronic diseases

13. _____ cultural competence

14. _____ energy density

15. _____ energy-yielding nutrients

16. _____ essential nutrients

17. _____ ethnic foods

18. _____ functional foods

19. _____ nutritional genomics

20. _____ phytochemicals

a. diseases characterized by slow progression and long duration, e.g., heart disease, diabetes, and some cancers

b. foods associated with particular cultural groups.

c. having an awareness and acceptance of cultures and the ability to interact effectively with people of diverse cultures

d. foods that contain bioactive components that provide health benefits beyond their nutrient contributions

e. nonnutrient compounds found in plants

f. nutrients a person must obtain from food because the body cannot make them for itself in sufficient quantity to meet physiological needs

g. the nutrients that break down to yield energy the body can use

h. units by which energy is measured

i. a measure of the energy a food provides relative to the weight of the food (kcalories per gram)

j. the science of how nutrients affect the activities of genes and how genes affect the interactions between diet and disease

21. _____ anthropometric

22. _____ Dietary Reference Intakes (DRI)

23. _____ malnutrition

24. _____ nutrition assessment

25. _____ overnutrition

26. _____ primary deficiency

27. _____ requirement

28. _____ risk factor

29. _____ secondary deficiency

30. _____ undernutrition

a. a set of nutrient intake values for healthy people in the United States and Canada

b. the lowest continuing intake of a nutrient that will maintain a specified criterion of adequacy

c. any condition caused by excess or deficient food energy or nutrient intake or by an imbalance of nutrients

d. deficient energy or nutrients

e. excess energy or nutrients

f. a comprehensive analysis of a person's nutrition status that uses health, socioeconomic, drug, and diet histories; anthropometric measurements; physical examinations; and laboratory tests

g. relating to measurement of the physical characteristics of the body, such as height and weight

h. a nutrient deficiency caused by inadequate dietary intake of a nutrient

i. a nutrient deficiency caused by something other than an inadequate intake such as a disease condition or drug interaction that reduces absorption, accelerates use, hastens excretion, or destroys the nutrient

j. a condition or behavior associated with an elevated frequency of a disease but not proved to be causal

Sample Test Questions

Select the best answer for each question.

1. When people eat foods associated with their families and geographical location, their eating patterns are being influenced by:
   a. personal preference.
   b. habit.
   c. ethnic heritage or tradition.
   d. physical appearance.
   e. nutrition.

2. People who eat foods to relieve boredom or calm anxiety are eating for reasons of:
   a. availability.
   b. nutrition.
   c. values.
   d. emotional comfort.
   e. economy.

3. To make food choices to improve health, people will:
   a. select foods that taste bad to them but are nutritious.
   b. consume only "special" foods that are expensive.
   c. purchase and eat only vegetables.
   d. be mindful of nutrition when making food choices.

4. A complete chemical analysis of your body would show that it is composed mostly of:
   a. proteins.
   b. carbohydrates.
   c. fats.
   d. water.
   e. minerals.

5. An organic compound is:
   a. a compound that contains carbon and hydrogen atoms.
   b. any substance found in living organisms.
   c. a compound that contains oxygen atoms.
   d. found only in foods grown under special conditions.
   e. superior.

6. Among these classes of nutrients, which one is not organic?
   a. Carbohydrate
   b. Fat
   c. Protein
   d. Vitamins
   e. Minerals

7. Which of the following does not yield energy for human use?
   a. Carbohydrates
   b. Vitamins
   c. Fats
   d. Proteins

8. When energy nutrients are metabolized:
   a. the arrangement of atoms remains unaltered.
   b. energy is released.
   c. the bonds between the nutrients' atoms break.
   d. a and b
   e. b and c

9. A kcalorie is a:
   a. gram of fat.
   b. unit in which energy is measured.
   c. heating device.
   d. term used to describe the amount of sugar and fat in foods.

10. Alcohol provides kcalories and
    a. is not considered a nutrient.
    b. sustains life.
    c. is useful for growth.
    d. promotes health.

11. A carbohydrate-rich food like bread:
    a. contains a mixture of the three energy nutrients.
    b. contains no protein.
    c. contains no protein or fat.
    d. cannot be properly classified on the basis of nutrient content.

12. One gram of alcohol provides:
    a. 4 kcal.
    b. 7 kcal.
    c. 9 kcal.
    d. 0 kcal.

8

13. Which of the following are vulnerable to destruction by heat and light?
    a. Carbohydrates
    b. Fats
    c. Vitamins
    d. Proteins
    e. Minerals

14. Minerals are:
    a. energy providers.
    b. indestructible.
    c. large.
    d. organic elements.

15. Water:
    a. is organic.
    b. gives us energy.
    c. is indispensable.
    d. is not a nutrient.

16. The science of nutrition is the study of:
    a. how to prepare delicious foods that will improve a person's health.
    b. the substances in foods, such as nutrients.
    c. the processes by which the body handles nutrients.
    d. a and b
    e. b and c

17. What type of research study observes how much and what kinds of foods a group of people eat?
    a. Human intervention
    b. Animal
    c. Case-control
    d. Epidemiological

18. The _____ are a set of four nutrient intake values that can be used to plan and evaluate diets for healthy people.
    a. RDA
    b. AI
    c. UL
    d. DRI

19. The dietary recommendations apply to:
    a. average daily intakes.
    b. healthy people.
    c. all people.
    d. a and b
    e. a and c

20. Historical information, physical examination, laboratory tests, and anthropometric measures are:
    a. steps in the scientific method.
    b. methods used in nutrition assessment.
    c. procedures used to determine the nutrient content of a diet.
    d. obsolete procedures used by nutritionists years ago.

21. A deficiency caused by an inadequate intake of a nutrient is a _____ deficiency.
    a. primary
    b. secondary
    c. dire
    d. clinical
    e. subclinical

22. A technique to detect nutrient deficiencies by taking height and weight measurements is part of the nutrition assessment component known as:
    a. diet history.
    b. anthropometrics.
    c. physical examination.
    d. biochemical tests.

23. Factors associated with elevated frequency of a disease but not proved to be causal are:
    a. medical factors.
    b. individual interventions.
    c. risk factors.
    d. disease clusters.

24. A research study often involves testing a(n):
    a. anecdote.
    b. sample size.
    c. validity.
    d. hypothesis.

25. A group that is not given the treatment is called the
    a. placebo.
    b. control group.
    c. experimental group.
    d. randomized group.

26. Which of the following is used to control for the placebo effect?
    a. Large sample size
    b. Blind experiment
    c. Positive correlation
    d. Randomization

27. A correlation between variables indicates that the:
    a. variables are associated.
    b. variables are causative.
    c. variables have a causative mechanism.
    d. All of the above

28. What process occurs when scientists evaluate studies for publication potential?
    a. Validity assessment
    b. Replication
    c. Experimental review
    d. Peer review

29. The average dietary energy intake required to maintain energy balance in a person who has a healthy body weight and level of physical activity is the:
    a. Tolerable Upper Intake Level (UL).
    b. Recommended Dietary Allowance (RDA).
    c. Estimated Energy Requirement (EER).
    d. Adequate Intake (AI).

30. According to the Acceptable Macronutrient Distribution Ranges (AMDR), the appropriate percentages of kcalories from carbohydrate, protein, and fat are:
    a. 35-45% carbohydrate, 20-35% fat, and 20-45% protein.
    b. 45-65% carbohydrate, 20-35% fat, and 10-35% protein.
    c. 45-65% carbohydrate, 10-25% fat, and 20-45% protein.
    d. 50-75% carbohydrate, 5-20% fat, and 10-35% protein.

31. Which of the following is true about recommendations?
    a. They are minimal requirements.
    b. They are optimal intakes for all individuals.
    c. They can target most people.
    d. They can account for individual variations in nutrient needs.

Short Answer Questions

1. Ten factors that influence food choices are:

   a.   f.

   b.   g.

   c.   h.

   d.   i.

   e.   j.

2. The six classes of nutrients are:

   a.   d.

   b.   e.

   c.   f.

3. The organic nutrients are:

   a.   c.

   b.   d.

4. The inorganic nutrients are:

   a.   b.

5. The nutrients that provide energy are:

   a.   c.

   b.

6. 1 gram carbohydrate   = _____ kcalories

   1 gram fat   = _____ kcalories

   1 gram protein   = _____ kcalories

   1 gram alcohol   = _____ kcalories

7. ½ cup vegetables   = _____ mL or _____ grams

   1 cup juice or milk   = _____ mL

8. The steps of the scientific method are:

   a.   c.

   b.   d.

9. The four categories of the Dietary Reference Intakes (DRI) are:

   a.

   b.

   c.

   d.

10. Name and describe the methods used in nutrition assessment.

    a.

    b.

    c.

    d.

11. The ten leading causes of death in the United States are:

    a.   f.

    b.   g.

    c.   h.

    d.   i.

    e.   j.

12. Nine factors contributing to deaths in the United States include:

a.   f.

b.   g.

c.   h.

d.   i.

e.

Problem Solving

1.   How many grams of fat were consumed if a person received 405 kcalories from fat in a day?

2.   How many kcalories are provided by 13 grams of carbohydrate?

3.   How many total kcalories are in 10 grams of carbohydrate, 4 grams of protein, 6 grams of fat, and 7 grams of alcohol?

4.   If a food product contains 20 grams of protein, how many kcalories will be provided from protein?

5.   If a food item contains 10 grams of protein and another food item contains 10 grams of carbohydrate, how many kcalories are provided from each and which item is more fattening?

6.   If an alcoholic beverage contains 1 gram of ethanol and 10 grams of carbohydrate, how many kcalories does it provide?

7.   A person consumes 100 grams of fat, 50 grams of carbohydrate, 30 grams of protein, 20 milligrams of the vitamin thiamin, and 250 milligrams of the mineral calcium. How much energy will this provide?

8.   A woman consumed 500 grams of carbohydrate, 30 grams of protein, and 75 grams of fat in one day. How many total kcalories did this provide, and how many and what percentage of kcalories were from carbohydrate, protein, and fat?

9.   A person consumed 400 grams of carbohydrate, 150 grams of protein, 300 grams of fat and 5 grams of ethanol in one day. How many total kcalories were provided, and how many and what percent of kcalories were from carbohydrate, protein, fat, and alcohol?

10. Meal A provides 250 grams of protein and 40 grams of fat. Meal B provides 250 grams of carbohydrate and 40 grams of fat. How many kcalories are provided by each meal?

❦ Chapter 1 Answer Key ❧

Summing Up

1. reasons
2. health
3. healthfulness
4. important
5. food
6. nutrients
7. maintenance
8. carbohydrates
9. minerals
10. energy-yielding
11. materials
12. energy
13. kcalories
14. water
15. experiments
16. experimental
17. large
18. placebos
19. replicated
20. evaluate
21. half
22. healthy
23. RDA
24. average
25. proportions
26. highest
27. malnourished
28. malnutrition
29. assessment
30. historical
31. earliest
32. anthropometric
33. populations
34. genetics
35. closely
36. choices

Chapter Study Questions

1. Preferences, habit, ethnic heritage or tradition, social interactions, availability, convenience, economy, positive and negative associations, emotional comfort, values, body weight and image, nutrition and health reasons.

2. The number one reason people choose certain foods is preferences, or taste—they like the flavor. To learn to select foods that provide nutrition and health benefits, people must be aware of the other influences on their food choices. Additionally, they need to know that they don't need to purchase any "special" foods to enjoy a healthy diet. They must be educated about nutrition and be mindful of nutrition when making selections.

3. A nutrient is a substance obtained from food and used in the body to promote growth, maintenance, and repair. Carbohydrate, fat, protein, vitamins, minerals, and water are the six nutrient classes. An essential nutrient is one that must be obtained from an outside source because the body cannot make it in a sufficient quantity to meet physiological needs.

4. Organic nutrients: carbohydrates, fats, proteins, vitamins. Inorganic nutrients: minerals, water. Organic literally means "alive" and refers to substances or molecules containing carbon-carbon bonds or carbon-hydrogen bonds, not necessarily living things. The inorganic nutrients do not contain carbon.

5. Energy-yielding nutrients: carbohydrate (4 kcal/g), fat (9 kcal/g), protein (4 kcal/g). Energy is measured in calories or kilocalories—a measure of heat energy.

6. In addition to providing energy, carbohydrates, proteins, and fats provide the raw materials for building the body's tissues and regulating its many activities. Proteins are found in structures such as the muscles and skin and help to regulate digestion and energy metabolism.

7. Alcohol yields energy (7 kcal per gram) when metabolized, but alcohol is not considered a nutrient because it does not support the growth, maintenance, or repair of the body.

8. The science of nutrition is the study of the nutrients and other substances in foods and the body's handling of them. Its foundation depends on several other sciences including biology, biochemistry, and physiology. Nutritional genomics is the science of how nutrients affect the activities of genes and how genes affect the interactions between diet and disease.

9. The scientific method begins with observation and a research question. A hypothesis (prediction) is developed to answer the question, and an experiment is designed to test the hypothesis. Once results are obtained, they are interpreted as either supporting or not supporting the hypothesis.

10. Epidemiological studies including cross-sectional, case-control, and cohort studies; and experimental studies including animal studies, in vitro studies, and human intervention (or clinical) trials are all used to acquire scientific information.

11. Correlations between variables indicate that they are associated with each other (change together); causal associations between variables require a known mechanism and indicate that one causes the other. Positive correlations indicate that as one increases, the other also increases. Negative correlations indicate that the variables change in opposite directions (as one increases, the other decreases).

12. The DRI are the Dietary Reference Intakes. They are a set of four nutrient intake values that can be used to plan and evaluate diets for healthy people. They are developed by the DRI Committee. Members of the committee are selected from the Food and Nutrition Board of the Institute of Medicine, the National Academy of Sciences, and Health Canada. They apply to healthy people in the U.S. and Canada.

13. The four categories include the Estimated Average Requirement (defines the amount of a nutrient that supports a specific function in the body for half of the population); the Recommended Dietary Allowance (uses Estimated Average Requirement to establish a goal for dietary intake that will meet the needs of almost all healthy people); the Adequate Intake (serves a similar purpose when an RDA cannot be determined); and the Tolerable Upper Intake Level (establishes the highest amount that appears safe for regular consumption).

14. How much of a nutrient a person needs, which is determined by studying deficiency states, nutrient stores, and depletion, and by measuring the body's intake and excretion of the nutrient; that different individuals have different requirements; at what dividing line the bulk of the population is covered.

15. When a person doesn't consume enough or consumes too much of a specific nutrient or energy over time, they get sick and show signs of deficiencies or excesses. Malnutrition is poor nutrition status, undernutrition is underconsumption of food energy or nutrients severe enough to cause disease or increased susceptibility to disease, and overnutrition is overconsumption of food energy or nutrients severe enough to cause disease or to cause increased susceptibility to disease. They are detected through nutrition assessment techniques (anthropometric measures, lab tests, physical findings, and diet history).

16. Administering questionnaires, conducting interviews, collecting anthropometric measurements, and conducting physical examinations on groups of people are methods used in nutrition surveys. Food consumption surveys and nutrition status surveys can provide information regarding amounts and kinds of foods people consume as well as evaluate people's nutrition status.

17. Factors that increase the risk of developing chronic diseases are called risk factors. A strong association between a risk factor and a disease means that when the factor is present, the likelihood of developing the disease increases. Common risk factors for disease include use of tobacco products, consuming a high-saturated fat diet, being overweight, having high blood pressure, being physically inactive, and having high blood cholesterol.

18. Risk factors tend to persist over time. Without intervention, people usually continue practicing the same behaviors from childhood into adulthood. Risk factors cluster; that is, people tend to practice more than one negative behavior at a time. Risk factors have different levels of influence on health—tobacco use is one of the strongest risk factors for disease. Despite the knowledge Americans have gained about the relationship between health and disease, they continue to practice negative behaviors.

14

Key Terms Practice

1. energy	9. nutrients	17. b	25. e
2. deficient	10. vitamins	18. d	26. h
3. minerals	11. h	19. j	27. b
4. inorganic	12. a	20. e	28. j
5. organic	13. c	21. g	29. i
6. nutrition	14. i	22. a	30. d
7. foods	15. g	23. c	
8. diet	16. f	24. f	

Sample Test Questions

1. c (p. 4)	9. b (p. 8)	17. d (p. 14)	25. b (p. 12)
2. d (p. 5)	10. a (p. 9)	18. d (p. 17)	26. b (p. 15)
3. d (p. 6)	11. a (p. 10)	19. d (p. 20)	27. a (p. 16)
4. d (pp. 6-7)	12. b (p. 9)	20. b (p. 22)	28. d (p. 16)
5. a (p. 7)	13. c (p. 11)	21. a (p. 23)	29. c (p. 20)
6. e (p. 7)	14. b (p. 11)	22. b (p. 22)	30. b (p. 20)
7. b (p. 8)	15. c (p. 11)	23. c (p. 26)	31. c (p. 20)
8. e (p. 10)	16. e (p. 12)	24. d (p. 12)	

Short Answer Questions

1. preferences; habit; ethnic heritage and regional cuisines; social interactions; availability (convenience and economy); positive and negative associations; emotions; values; body weight and image; nutrition and health benefits

2. carbohydrate; fat; protein; vitamins; minerals; water

3. carbohydrate; fat; protein; vitamins

4. minerals; water

5. carbohydrate; fat; protein

6. carbohydrate = 4; fat = 9; protein = 4; alcohol = 7

7. vegetables = 120 mL or 100 g; liquid = 240 mL

8. observation and question; hypothesis and prediction; experiment; results and interpretations

9. Estimated Average Requirements (EAR); Recommended Dietary Allowances (RDA); Adequate Intakes (AI); Tolerable Upper Intake Levels (UL)

10. historical information – consult person or medical records regarding family, situation, and prior health status and collect information about foods eaten over a period of time; anthropometric measures – measure height, weight, body parts; physical examination – inspect body parts (hair, eyes, skin); laboratory tests – analyze body samples (blood, urine)

11. heart disease; cancers; chronic lung diseases; strokes; accidents; Alzheimer's disease; diabetes mellitus; pneumonia and influenza; kidney disease; suicide

12. tobacco; poor diet/inactivity; alcohol; microbial agents; toxic agents; motor vehicles; firearms; sexual behavior; illicit drugs

Problem Solving

1. 45 g (405 kcal divided by 9 kcal/g fat = 45 g fat)

2. 52 kcal (13 g carb multiplied by 4 kcal/g carb = 52 kcal)

3. 159 kcal (10 g carb × 4 kcal/g + 4 g pro × 4 kcal/g + 6 g fat × 9 kcal/g + 7 g alc × 7 kcal/g = 40 + 16 + 54 + 49 = 159 kcal)

4. 20 g × 4 = 80 kcalories from protein

5. 10 g × 4 = 40 kcalories from protein
   10 g × 4 = 40 kcalories from carbohydrate
   They each provide 40 kcalories and they are equally fattening.

6. 1 g ethanol × 7 = 7 kcalories from ethanol
   10 g carb × 4 = 40 kcalories from carbohydrate
   7 + 40 = 47 kcalories

7. 100 g fat × 9 = 900 kcalories from fat
   50 g carb × 4 = 200 kcalories from carbohydrate
   30 g protein × 4 = 120 kcalories from protein
   20 mg thiamin = 0 kcalories
   250 mg calcium = 0 kcalories
   900 + 200 + 120 = 1220 total kcalories

8. 500 g carbohydrate × 4 = 2000 kcal
   30 g protein × 4 = 120 kcal
   75 g fat × 9 = 675 kcal
   2000 + 120 + 675 = 2795 total kcalories
   2000/2795 = 72% kcalories from carbohydrate
   120/2795 = 4% kcalories from protein
   675/2795 = 24% kcalories from fat

9. 400 g carbohydrate × 4 = 1600 kcalories
   150 g protein × 4 = 600 kcalories
   300 g fat × 9 = 2700 kcalories
   5 g ethanol × 7 = 35 kcalories
   1600 + 600 + 2700 + 35 = 4935 total kcalories
   1600/4935 = 32% kcalories from carbohydrate
   600/4935 = 12% kcalories from protein
   2700/4935 = 55% kcalories from fat
   35/4935 = 1% kcalories from ethanol

10. Meal A: 250 g protein × 4 = 1000 kcal; 40 g fat × 9 = 360 kcal; 1000 + 360 = 1360 kcalories
    Meal B: 250 g carbohydrate × 4 = 1000 kcal; 40 g fat × 9 = 360 kcal; 1000 + 360 = 1360 kcalories
    They provide the same number of kcalories.

✆ Chapter 2 ~ Planning a Healthy Diet ✆

Chapter Outline

I. Principles and Guidelines
    A. Diet-Planning Principles
        1. Adequacy
        2. Balance
        3. kCalorie (Energy) Control
        4. Nutrient Density
        5. Moderation
        6. Variety
    B. *Dietary Guidelines for Americans*
II. Diet-Planning Guides
    A. USDA Food Patterns
        1. Recommended Amounts
        2. Notable Nutrients
        3. Nutrient-Dense Choices
        4. Discretionary kCalories
        5. Serving Equivalents
        6. Ethnic Food Choices
        7. Vegetarian Food Guide
        8. Mixtures of Foods
        9. MyPlate
        10. Recommendations versus Actual
             Intakes
        11. MyPlate Shortcomings
    B. Exchange Lists
    C. Putting the Plan into Action
    D. From Guidelines to Groceries
        1. Grains
        2. Vegetables
        3. Fruit
        4. Protein Foods
        5. Milk and Milk Products
III. Food Labels
    A. The Ingredient List
    B. Nutrition Facts Panel
        1. Serving Sizes
        2. Nutrient Quantities
        3. The Daily Values
    C. Claims on Labels
        1. Nutrient Claims
        2. Health Claims
        3. Structure-Function Claims
    D. Consumer Education
IV. Vegetarian Diets
    A. Health Benefits of Vegetarian Diets
        1. Obesity
        2. Diabetes
        3. Hypertension
        4. Heart Disease
        5. Cancer
        6. Other Diseases
    B. Vegetarian Diet Planning
        1. Protein
        2. Iron
        3. Zinc
        4. Calcium
        5. Vitamin B_{12}
        6. Vitamin D
        7. Omega-3 Fatty Acids
    C. Healthy Food Choices

Summing Up

A well-planned diet delivers 1._____ nutrients, a 2._____ array of nutrients, and an appropriate amount of 3._____. It is based on 4._____-_____ foods, moderate in substances that can be 5._____ to health, and 6._____ in its selections. The 7._____ _____ apply these principles, offering practical 8._____ on how to eat for good health.

Food group plans such as the USDA 9._____ _____ help consumers select the types and 10._____ of foods to provide 11._____, balance, and 12._____ in the diet. They make it easier to plan a diet that includes a balance of grains, 13._____, fruits, protein foods, and 14._____ products. In making any food choice, remember to view the food in the context of the 15._____ diet. The 16._____ of many different foods provides the array of nutrients that is so essential to a 17._____ diet.

Food 18._____ provide consumers with information they need to 19._____ foods that will help them meet their nutrition and health 20._____. When labels contain 21._____ information presented in a 22._____, easy-to-read format, consumers are well prepared to 23._____ and create healthful diets.

Chapter Study Questions

1. Name the diet-planning principles and briefly describe how each principle helps in diet planning.

2. What key recommendations appear in the *Dietary Guidelines for Americans*?

3. Name the five food groups used in the USDA Food Patterns and identify several foods typical of each group. Explain how these patterns group foods, and how they incorporate the concepts of nutrient density and kcalorie control.

4. Review the *Dietary Guidelines*. What types of grocery selections would you make to achieve those recommendations?

5. Define the terms *nutrient density* and *discretionary kcalorie allowance*. Which foods provide the "notable nutrients" most often lacking in the American diet?

6. Describe the purpose of MyPlate.

7. Discuss how exchange lists are used in diet planning.

18

8. What information can you expect to find on a food label? How can this information help you choose between two similar products?

9. What are the Daily Values? How can they help you meet health recommendations?

10. List and define the three types of claims that may be on a food product.

Key Terms Practice

To complete the crossword puzzle, identify the key term that best matches each definition.

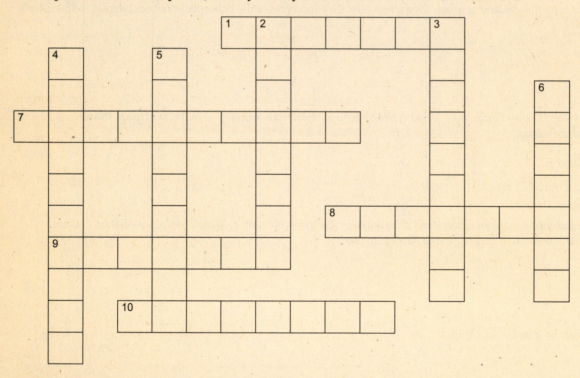

Across:
1. Plants of the bean and pea family, with seeds that are rich in protein compared with other plant-derived foods.
7. Providing enough but not too much of a substance.
8. Providing foods in proportion to one another and in proportion to the body's needs.
9. The process by which the coarse parts of a food are removed. When wheat is refined into flour, the bran, germ, and husk are removed, leaving only the endosperm.
10. Providing all the essential nutrients, fiber, and energy in amounts sufficient to maintain health.

Down:

2. The addition to a food of specific nutrients to replace losses that occur during processing so that the food will meet a specified standard.
3. Fats that are not usually liquid at room temperature; commonly found in most foods derived from animals and vegetable oils that have been hydrogenated.
4. A grain that maintains the same relative proportions of starchy endosperm, germ, and bran as the original (all but the husk).
5. The addition to a food of nutrients that were either not originally present or present in insignificant amounts.
6. Characterized by eating a wide selection of foods within and among the major food groups.

Match the key terms with their definitions.

11. _____ added sugars

12. _____ discretionary kcalories

13. _____ eating pattern

14. _____ empty-kcalorie foods

15. _____ food group plans

16. _____ kcalorie control

17. _____ nutrient density

18. _____ nutrient profiling

19. _____ portion sizes

20. _____ serving sizes

a. customary intake of foods and beverages over time
b. management of food energy intake
c. a measure of the nutrients a food provides relative to the energy it provides
d. a popular term used to denote foods that contribute energy but lack protein, vitamins, and minerals
e. ranking foods based on their nutrient composition
f. sugars and other kcaloric sweeteners that are added to foods during processing, preparation, or at the table
g. diet-planning tools that sort foods into groups based on nutrient content and then specify that people should eat certain amounts of foods from each group
h. the kcalories remaining in a person's energy allowance after consuming enough nutrient-dense foods to meet all nutrient needs for a day
i. the standardized quantity of a food; such information allows comparisons when reading food labels and consistency when following the *Dietary Guidelines*
j. the quantity of a food served or eaten at one meal or snack; not a standard amount.

21. _____ Daily Values (DV)

22. _____ exchange lists

23. _____ food substitutes

24. _____ health claims

25. _____ imitation foods

26. _____ nutrient claims

27. _____ percent Daily Value (%DV)

28. _____ processed foods

29. _____ structure-function claims

30. _____ textured vegetable protein

a. diet-planning tools that organize foods by their proportions of carbohydrate, fat, and protein
b. foods that have been treated to change their physical, chemical, microbiological, or sensory properties
c. processed soybean protein used in vegetarian products such as soy burgers
d. foods that substitute for and resemble another food, but are nutritionally inferior to it with respect to vitamin, mineral, or protein content
e. foods that are designed to replace other foods
f. reference values developed by the FDA specifically for use on food labels
g. the percentage of a Daily Value recommendation found in a specified serving of food for key nutrients based on a 2000-kcalorie diet
h. statements that characterize the quantity of a nutrient in a food
i. statements that characterize the relationship between a nutrient or other substance in a food and a disease or health-related condition
j. statements that characterize the relationship between a nutrient or other substance in a food and its role in the body

Sample Test Questions

Select the best answer for each question.

1. Diet planning principles include:
   a. adequacy, B vitamins, carbohydrates, moderation, nutrient density, and variety.
   b. abundance, balance, carbohydrates, meals, nutrients, and vegetables.
   c. adequacy, balance, kcalorie control, nutrient density, moderation, and variety.
   d. abundance, B vitamins, kcalorie control, milk, moderation, and vegetables.

2. Selecting foods that deliver the most nutrients for the least food energy is applying the concept of:
   a. moderation.
   b. abundance.
   c. variety.
   d. adequacy.
   e. nutrient density.

3. Which of the following is the most nutrient-dense food relative to calcium content?
   a. Whole milk
   b. Non-fat milk
   c. Low-fat milk
   d. Cheddar cheese

4. Foods that are low in nutrient density are:
   a. empty-kcalorie foods.
   b. raw vegetables.
   c. those that deliver protein, vitamins, and minerals with few kcalories.
   d. low in fat and sugar.

5. Key topics that are part of the *Dietary Guidelines for Americans*' recommendations include:
   a. foods and food components to reduce.
   b. balancing kcalories to manage weight.
   c. building healthy eating patterns.
   d. All of the above

6. An adult following the USDA Food Patterns should consume a variety of vegetables from all _____ subgroups of vegetables each week.
   a. one
   b. two
   c. three
   d. four
   e. five

7. Which of the following is descriptive of the USDA Food Patterns?
   a. A figure designed to assist the average consumer in the use of the Food Exchange System
   b. An educational tool for teaching nutrition to children that consists of food blocks that require stacking in a specific order
   c. A system that assigns foods to five major groups and recommends daily amounts of foods from each group
   d. A system of specialized containers of several different sizes which allows for better storage and preservation of perishable food items

8. The USDA Food Patterns categorize foods into the following major groups:
   a. fruits, vegetables, grains, protein foods, and milk/milk products.
   b. fruits, vegetables, grains, protein foods, and oils.
   c. fruits and vegetables, breads, meats, fats, and carbohydrate.
   d. fruits and vegetables, breads, meats, legumes, and dairy.

9. Exchange lists group foods according to:
   1. protein, fat, and carbohydrate content.
   2. water content.
   3. vitamin content.
   4. mineral content.

   a. 1 only
   b. 2 only
   c. 3 and 4
   d. 1, 2, 3, and 4

10. The USDA Food Patterns divide the vegetable group into 5 subgroups for the following reason:
   a. these groups each provide a different assortment of fats.
   b. people were consuming too many legumes.
   c. the vegetable group is widely enjoyed.
   d. some vegetables are especially good sources of certain nutrients.

11. The USDA Food Patterns encourage consumption of foods that provide "notable nutrients," meaning:
   a. nutrients that are needed in greater amounts than other nutrients.
   b. nutrients that have more important body functions than other nutrients.
   c. nutrients that are contained in empty-kcalorie foods.
   d. nutrients most often lacking in the diets of Americans.

12. The difference between kcalories needed to supply nutrients and those needed for energy is:
   a. nutrient density kcalories.
   b. notable nutrient kcalories.
   c. discretionary kcalories.
   d. empty kcalories.

13. A USDA educational tool that illustrates the food groups is called:
   a. the Exchange Lists.
   b. the *Healthy People 2020* objectives.
   c. MyPlate.
   d. the Sample Diet Plan.

14. Which of the following is characteristic of the USDA Food Patterns?
   a. They are used primarily by diabetics.
   b. They define food portions according to energy content.
   c. The groupings are made according to nutrient content.
   d. They subdivide the grain group based on fiber content.

15. What is the recommendation regarding grain products?
   a. Consume 3 whole-grain products per day.
   b. At least half should be whole grains.
   c. Eat 6 enriched products a day.
   d. Take 2 tablespoons of laxatives each day.

16. Which of the following is a characteristic of enriched grain products?
   a. They have all of the added nutrients listed on the label.
   b. They have the fiber restored from the refining procedure.
   c. They have 4 vitamins and 4 minerals added by the food processor.
   d. They have virtually all the nutrients restored from the refining procedure.

17. Suppose you are shopping for grains. Which type of product is rich in all nutrients found in the original grain?
   a. Refined
   b. Enriched
   c. Whole grain
   d. Fiber rich

18. Dried beans and peas, pinto beans, lima beans, and black beans are examples of:
   a. legumes.
   b. meats.
   c. milk alternatives.
   d. fruits.

19. Whole-grain bread contains more of the following nutrients than enriched bread:
   a. iron, carbohydrate, and protein.
   b. iron, thiamin, riboflavin, and niacin.
   c. magnesium, zinc, fiber, and vitamin B_6.
   d. water, fiber, and fat.

20. Corn, green peas, and potatoes are listed with breads in which food plan?
    a. USDA Food Patterns
    b. Exchange lists
    c. Healthy Eating Index
    d. Four food group plan

21. Foods that substitute for and resemble another food but are nutritionally inferior to it are called:
    a. functional foods.
    b. food substitutes.
    c. food density.
    d. imitation foods.

22. Another name for fat-free milk is:
    a. nonfat milk.
    b. low-fat milk.
    c. reduced-fat milk.
    d. less-fat milk.

23. Wise consumers will take this action before using soy products as substitutes for dairy:
    a. check expiration dates.
    b. read labels to determine the cholesterol and saturated fat contents.
    c. check to see if they are organic.
    d. read labels to see if they have been fortified with vitamins B_{12} and D and calcium.

24. The items on a food label that tell consumers about the nutritional value of a product include:
    1. the common or usual name of the product.
    2. the net contents in terms of weight, measure, or count.
    3. the ingredients in descending order of predominance.
    4. the serving size and number of servings per container.
    5. the quantities of specified nutrients and food constituents.

    a. 1, 2, 3, and 4
    b. 2, 3, 4, and 5
    c. 3, 4, and 5
    d. All of the above

25. The serving size on a label:
    a. varies according to brand.
    b. is set at 8 fluid ounces for all beverages.
    c. is set at 1 cup for all ice creams.
    d. b and c

26. The FDA uses _____ kcalories as a standard for energy intake in calculating the Daily Values (DV) for energy-yielding nutrients.
    a. 1,200
    b. 1,500
    c. 1,800
    d. 2,000

27. If you see "good source of fiber" on a label, this is an example of:
    a. a nutrient claim.
    b. a health claim.
    c. a structure-function claim.
    d. All of the above

28. If you see "Diets low in sodium may reduce the risk of high blood pressure," on a label, this is an example of:
    a. a nutrient claim.
    b. a health claim.
    c. a structure-function claim.
    d. All of the above

29. If you read, "builds strong bones," on a label, this is an example of:
    a. a nutrient claim.
    b. a health claim.
    c. a structure-function claim.
    d. All of the above

30. If a food product provides between 10 and 19 percent of the Daily Value for a nutrient, the food is considered a _____ source.
    a. high
    b. excellent
    c. good
    d. low

31. Statements that characterize the relationship between a nutrient or other substance in a food and its role in the body are:
    a. health claims.
    b. nutrient claims.
    c. structure-function claims.
    d. All of the above

Short Answer Questions

1. Diet-planning principles include:

   a.   d.

   b.   e.

   c.   f.

2. The four major topic areas of the *Dietary Guidelines* include:

   a.

   b.

   c.

   d.

3. The two types of diet-planning guides most widely used are:

   a.   b.

4. The five major groups in the USDA Food Patterns are:

   a.   d.

   b.   e.

   c.

5. The five vegetable subgroups are:

   a.   d.

   b.   e.

   c.

6. The three protein foods subgroups are:

   a.   c.

   b.

7. Three general types of information shown in the Nutrition Facts panel on a food label are:

   a.   c.

   b.

8. Three types of claims that may be found on food labels are:

   a.   c.

   b.

Problem Solving

1. Using the exchange system (Appendix G), how many kcalories are in the following breakfast?

    1 slice of whole-wheat toast with
    1 tsp butter
    1 small banana, ½ cup apple juice
    1 ½ cups nonfat milk

2. A food item provides 400 mg of calcium and has 350 kcalories. Calculate the nutrient density value.

3. One food item provides 10 mg of iron and 100 kcalories. Another food item provides 15 mg of iron and 175 kcalories. Calculate the nutrient density for both food items. Which is a better choice?

4. A recipe calls for 2 teaspoons of sugar. Calculate this amount in milliliters (mL).

5. You are trying to consume 8 cups of water a day. How many milliliters (mL) is this?

6. Suppose your energy requirements are 2500 kcal per day. Calculate your personal Daily Value for g of fat per day.

7. Suppose your energy requirements are 1800 kcal per day. Calculate your personal Daily Value for g of fat per day.

8. Your friend's energy requirements are 3000 kcal per day. How many grams of carbohydrate, fiber, and protein would he require, based on personalized Daily Values? What is the maximum amount of saturated fat he should eat each day based on his personalized Daily Value?

9. The serving size for a food item is ¾ cup. You have consumed 3 cups. How many servings did you eat?

10. The serving size for a food item is ¾ cup and each serving has 120 kcalories. You have consumed 3 cups. How many kcalories did the food provide?

❧ Chapter 2 Answer Key ❧

Summing Up

1. adequate
2. balanced
3. energy
4. nutrient-dense
5. detrimental
6. varied
7. *Dietary Guidelines*
8. advice
9. Food Patterns
10. amounts
11. adequacy
12. variety
13. vegetables
14. milk
15. total
16. combination
17. healthy
18. labels
19. select
20. goals
21. relevant
22. standardized
23. plan

Chapter Study Questions

1. Adequacy—providing all essential nutrients. Balance—providing foods of a number of types in proportion to each other so that foods rich in some nutrients do not crowd out foods rich in other nutrients. Kilocalorie control—management of food energy intake. Nutrient density—selecting foods with high nutrient value relative to food energy. Moderation—providing enough but not too much of a dietary constituent. Variety—using different foods on different occasions; variety helps ensure adequacy and balance.

2. Prevent and/or reduce overweight and obesity through improved eating and physical activity behaviors. Control total kcalorie intake to manage body weight. Increase physical activity and reduce time spent in sedentary behaviors. Maintain appropriate kcalorie balance during each stage of life. Reduce daily sodium intake to less that 2300 milligrams and further reduce intake to 1500 milligrams among persons who are 51 and older and those of any age who are African American or have hypertension, diabetes, or chronic kidney disease. Consume less than 10 percent of kcalories from saturated fats by replacing them with monounsaturated and polyunsaturated fats. Consume less than 300 milligrams per day of dietary cholesterol. Keep *trans* fat consumption as low as possible by limiting foods that contain synthetic sources of *trans* fats, such as partially hydrogenated oils, and by limiting other solid fats. Reduce the intake of kcalories from solid fats and added sugars. Limit the consumption of foods that contain refined grains, especially refined grain foods that contain solid fats, added sugars, and sodium. If alcohol is consumed it should be consumed in moderation—up to one drink per day for women and two drinks per day for men—and only by adults of legal drinking age. Increase vegetable and fruit intake. Eat a variety of vegetables, especially dark-green and red and orange vegetables and legumes. Consume at least half of all grains as whole grains. Increase whole-grain intake by replacing refined grains with whole grains. Increase intake of fat-free or low-fat milk and milk products, such as milk, yogurt, cheese, or fortified soy beverages. Choose a variety of protein foods, which include seafood, lean meat and poultry, eggs, legumes, soy products, and unsalted nuts and seeds. Increase the amount and variety of seafood consumed by choosing seafood in place of some meat and poultry. Replace protein foods that are higher in solid fats with choices that are lower in solid fats and kcalories and/or are sources of oils. Use oils to replace solid fats where possible. Choose foods that provide more potassium, dietary fiber, calcium, and vitamin D. Select an eating pattern that meets nutrient needs over time at an appropriate kcalorie level. Account for all foods and beverages consumed and assess how they fit within a total healthy eating pattern. Follow food safety recommendations when preparing and eating foods to reduce the risk of foodborne illnesses.

3. See Figure 2-2 for food groups and foods typical of each group. The USDA Food Patterns group foods similar in origin and that make notable contributions of the same key nutrients. Nutrient density and kcalorie control are addressed in that the plan points out foods that are more and less nutrient dense and recommends quantities of the more nutrient-dense vegetables and protein foods to consume over the course of a week. The plan also gives specific recommended amounts of food to eat each day for people with different kcalorie needs, and limits for the discretionary kcalorie allowance (which is the maximum kcal allowed from energy-dense, nutrient-poor foods).

4. Start with the foods you regularly enjoy eating and then try to make a few improvements. For most people that will mean eating less red meats, cheeses, and salted snacks and more fruits, vegetables, whole grains, legumes, nuts, milk products, and seafood. When shopping, think of the food groups, and choose nutrient-dense foods within each group. Select more fresh foods and fewer processed foods. Add more whole grains to the diet; e.g.,

eat oatmeal for breakfast and popcorn for a snack or substitute brown rice for white rice and whole-wheat bread for enriched white bread.

Choose fresh vegetables often, especially dark green leafy and red and orange vegetables like spinach, broccoli, tomatoes, and sweet potatoes. Frozen and canned vegetables without added salt are acceptable alternatives to fresh. Choose often from the variety of legumes available. Choose fresh fruits often. Frozen, dried, and canned fruits without added sugar are acceptable alternatives to fresh. Choose lean cuts of beef and pork named "round" or "loin" (as in top round or pork tenderloin). As a guide, "prime" and "choice" cuts generally have more fat than "select" cuts.

Choose a variety of protein foods, which include seafood, lean meats and poultry, eggs, legumes, soy products, and unsalted nuts and seeds. Increase the amount and variety of seafood consumed by choosing seafood in place of some meat and poultry. Choose fat-free or low-fat milk, yogurt, and cheeses. Select milk to which vitamins A and D have been added and/or soy milk to which calcium, vitamin D, and vitamin B_{12} have been added. Select only soy beverages that have been fortified.

5. Nutrient density: a measure of the nutrients a food provides relative to the energy it provides; the more nutrients and fewer kcalories, the higher the nutrient density. Discretionary kcalorie allowance: the kcalories remaining in a person's energy allowance after consuming enough nutrient-dense foods to meet all nutrient needs for a day. Nutrients that are most often lacking in the diets of Americans, including fiber, vitamin D, calcium, and potassium, as well as other key nutrients such as vitamin A, vitamin C, vitamin E, and magnesium, can be obtained by eating plenty of dark green vegetables, orange vegetables, legumes, fruits, whole grains, seafood, and low-fat milk and milk products.

6. MyPlate is a diet planning educational program that can be used to remind consumers to consume a healthy diet. The MyPlate icon divides a plate into four sections, each representing a food group—fruits, vegetables, grains, and protein. The sections vary in size, indicating the relative proportion each food group contributes to a healthy diet. A circle next to the plate represents the milk group (dairy). MyPlate educates consumers about healthy food and physical activity choices, and it helps consumers choose the kinds and amounts of foods to eat each day. A key message of the website is to enjoy food but eat less by avoiding oversized portions.

7. Exchange lists are well suited to help a person achieve kcalorie control and moderation. Consumers can select foods from exchange lists that are significant to energy content. Originally developed for managing diabetes, exchange lists have proved useful for general diet planning as well. Exchange list sort foods according to their energy-nutrient contributions rather than their vitamin and mineral content.

8. The common or usual name of the product; the name and address of the manufacturer, packer, or distributor; the net contents in terms of weight, measure, or count; the ingredients in descending order of predominance by weight; the serving size and number of servings per container; and the quantities of specified nutrients and food constituents. Consumers can use the Nutrition Facts panel (especially the kcal and %DV) and ingredient lists to compare the nutrient densities and energy densities of products.

9. Daily Values are reference values developed by the FDA for use on food labels; they help people compare the nutrient contents of foods to recommended intakes and to the contents of other foods. Consumers can use the Daily Values to choose foods relatively low in detrimental constituents (e.g., saturated and *trans* fats) and high in beneficial ones (e.g., fiber or calcium).

10. Nutrient claims: statements that characterize the quantity of a nutrient in a food. Health claims: statements that characterize the relationship between a nutrient or other substance in a food and a disease or health-related condition. Structure-function claims: statements that characterize the relationship between a nutrient or other substance in a food and its role in the body.

Key Terms Practice

1. legumes	6. variety	11. f	16. b
2. enriched	7. moderation	12. h	17. c
3. solid fats	8. balance	13. a	18. e
4. whole grain	9. refined	14. d	19. j
5. fortified	10. adequacy	15. g	20. i

21. f	24. i	27. g	30. c
22. a	25. d	28. b	
23. e	26. h	29. j	

Sample Test Questions

1. c (pp. 36, 38)	9. a (p. 47)	17. c (p. 49)	25. b (p. 54)
2. e (p. 36)	10. d (pp. 40-41)	18. a (p. 52)	26. d (pp. 54, 55)
3. b (p. 36)	11. d (p. 41)	19. c (p. 51)	27. a (p. 56)
4. a (pp. 36, 38)	12. c (p. 44)	20. b (p. 47)	28. b (p. 57)
5. d (p. 39)	13. c (p. 45)	21. d (p. 53)	29. c (p. 57)
6. e (pp. 40-41)	14. c (p. 40)	22. a (p. 53)	30. c (pp. 56, 57)
7. c (p. 40)	15. b (p. 42)	23. d (p. 53)	31. c (pp. 57-58)
8. a (p. 40)	16. a (p. 49)	24. c (pp. 54-55)	

Short Answer Questions

1. adequacy, balance, kcalorie control, nutrient density, moderation, variety
2. balancing kcalories to manage weight; foods and food components to reduce; foods and nutrients to increase; building healthy eating patterns
3. food group plans *or* USDA Food Patterns, exchange systems
4. fruits, vegetables, grains, protein foods, milk and milk products
5. dark green vegetables, red and orange vegetables, legumes, starchy vegetables, other vegetables
6. seafood; meats, poultry, and eggs; nuts, seeds, and soy products
7. serving size, energy/nutrient quantities, Daily Values
8. nutrient claims, health claims, structure-function claims

Problem Solving

1. $80 + 45 + 2(60) + 1.5(100) = 395$ kcal

2. 400 mg calcium divided by 350 kcal = 1.14 mg calcium per kcalorie

3. 10 mg iron divided by 100 kcal = 0.1; 15 mg iron divided by 175 kcalories = .085.
   The first item has greater nutrient density, and based on this information is a better choice.

4. 2 teaspoons × 5 mL = 10 milliliters (mL)

5. 8 cups × 240 mL in a cup = 1920 milliliters (mL)

6. 2500 × 0.30 kcal from fat = 750 kcal divided by 9 kcal/g = 83 grams of fat

7. 1800 × 0.30 kcal from fat = 540 kcal divided by 9 kcal/g = 60 grams of fat

8. 3000 × 0.60 = 1800 kcal from carbohydrate; 1800 divided by 4 = 450 grams carbohydrate
   3000 divided by 1000 kcal = 3.0; 3.0 × 11.5 g = 34.5 grams fiber
   3000 × 0.10 = 300 kcal divided by 4 = 75 grams of protein
   3000 × 0.10 = 300 kcal from saturated fat; 300 kcal divided by 9 = 33 grams saturated fat per day

9. 3 cups divided by 0.75 cup per serving = 4 servings

10. 3 cups divided by 0.75 cup per serving = 4 servings × 120 kcalories = 480 kcalories

❻ Chapter 3 ~ Digestion, Absorption, and Transport ❸

Chapter Outline

I. Digestion
    A. Anatomy of the Digestive Tract
        1. Mouth
        2. Esophagus
        3. Stomach
        4. Small Intestine
        5. Large Intestine (Colon)
    B. The Muscular Action of Digestion
        1. Peristalsis
        2. Stomach Action
        3. Segmentation
        4. Sphincter Contractions
    C. The Secretions of Digestion
        1. Saliva
        2. Gastric Juice
        3. Pancreatic Juice and Intestinal Enzymes
        4. Bile
    D. The Final Stage
II. Absorption
    A. Anatomy of the Absorptive System
    B. A Closer Look at the Intestinal Cells
        1. Specialized Cells
        2. Food Combining

        3. Preparing Nutrients for Transport
III. The Circulatory Systems
    A. The Vascular System
    B. The Lymphatic System
IV. The Health and Regulation of the GI Tract
    A. Gastrointestinal Bacteria
    B. Gastrointestinal Hormones and Nerve Pathways
    C. The System at Its Best
V. Common Digestive Problems
    A. Choking
    B. Vomiting
    C. Diarrhea
        1. Irritable Bowel Syndrome
        2. Colitis
        3. Celiac Disease
        4. Treatment
    D. Constipation
    E. Belching and Gas
        1. Belching
        2. Intestinal Gas
    F. Gastroesophageal Reflux
    G. Ulcers

Summing Up

Food enters the mouth and travels down the 1._____ and through the upper and lower esophageal 2._____ to the stomach, then through the 3._____ sphincter to the small intestine, on through the 4._____ valve to the 5._____ _____, past the appendix to the 6._____, ending at the anus. The wavelike contractions of 7._____ and the periodic squeezing of 8._____ keep things moving at a reasonable pace. Along the way, secretions from the 9._____ glands, stomach, 10._____, liver (via the 11._____), and small intestine deliver fluids and 12._____ enzymes.

The many folds and 13._____ of the small intestine dramatically increase its 14._____ area, facilitating nutrient 15._____. Nutrients pass through the cells of the villi and enter either the 16._____ (if they are water soluble or small fat fragments) or the 17._____ (if they are fat soluble).

Nutrients leaving the 18._____ system via the blood are routed directly to the 19._____ before being transported to the body's 20._____. Those leaving via the 21._____ system (large fats and fat-soluble vitamins) eventually enter the vascular system but 22._____ the liver at first.

A diverse and abundant 23._____ population supports 24._____ health. The regulation of GI processes depends on the coordinated efforts of the 25._____ system and the nervous system. Together, digestion and 26._____ break down foods into 27._____ for the body's use. To function optimally, a healthy GI tract needs a 28._____ diet, adequate rest, and regular 29._____ activity.

Chapter Study Questions

1. Describe the challenges associated with digesting food and the solutions offered by the human body.

2. Describe the path food follows as it travels through the digestive system. Summarize the muscular actions that take place along the way.

3. Name five organs that secrete digestive juices. How do the juices and enzymes facilitate digestion?

4. Describe how the anatomy of the small intestine assists in nutrient absorption.

5. Discuss how different nutrients are absorbed into intestinal cells.

6. How is blood routed through the digestive system? Which nutrients enter the bloodstream directly? Which are first absorbed into the lymph?

7. Describe how the body coordinates and regulates the processes of digestion and absorption.

8. Discuss the role of gastrointestinal bacteria in maintaining the health of the GI tract.

9. How does the composition of the diet influence the functioning of the GI tract?

10. What steps can you take to help your GI tract function at its best?

Key Terms Practice

To complete the crossword puzzle, identify the key term that best matches each definition.

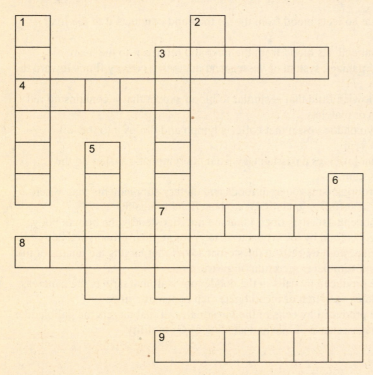

Across:

3. The semiliquid mass of partly digested food expelled by the stomach into the duodenum.
4. Bacteria in the intestines.
7. Milk product that results from the fermentation of lactic acid in milk by *Lactobacillus bulgaricus* and *Streptococcus thermophilus*.
8. A portion; with respect to food, the amount swallowed at one time.
9. Tubular glands that lie between the intestinal villi and secrete intestinal juices into the small intestine.

Down:

1. A backward flow.
2. The unit of measure expressing a substance's acidity or alkalinity.
3. A compound that facilitates chemical reactions without itself being changed in the process.
5. Fingerlike projections from the folds of the small intestine.
6. Waste matter discharged from the colon.

Match the key terms with their definitions.

10. _____ absorption

11. _____ digestion

12. _____ capillaries

13. _____ digestive system

14. _____ gastrointestinal tract

15. _____ goblet cells

16. _____ hepatic portal vein

17. _____ microvilli

18. _____ peristalsis

19. _____ segmentation

a. the process by which food is broken down into absorbable units

b. the uptake of nutrients by the cells of the small intestine for transport into either the blood or the lymph

c. the digestive tract

d. all the organs and glands associated with the ingestion and digestion of food

e. wavelike muscular contractions of the GI tract that push its contents along

f. a periodic squeezing or partitioning of the intestine at intervals along its length by its circular muscles

g. tiny, hairlike projections on each cell of every villus that can trap nutrient particles and transport them into the cells

h. cells of the GI tract (and lungs) that secrete mucus

i. small vessels that branch from an artery and connect arteries to veins; exchange of oxygen, nutrients, and waste materials takes place across their walls

j. the vein that collects blood from the GI tract and conducts it to the liver

20. _____ cholecystokinin

21. _____ gastrin

22. _____ hepatic vein

23. _____ lymph

24. _____ lymphatic system

25. _____ prebiotics

26. _____ probiotics

27. _____ secretin

28. _____ subclavian vein

29. _____ thoracic duct

a. the vein that collects blood from the liver and returns it to the heart

b. a loosely organized system of vessels and ducts that convey fluids toward the heart.

c. a clear yellowish fluid that is similar to blood except that it contains no red blood cells or platelets

d. the main lymphatic vessel that collects lymph and drains into the left subclavian vein

e. the vein that provides a passageway from the lymphatic system to the vascular system

f. living microorganisms found in foods and dietary supplements that, when consumed in sufficient quantities, are beneficial to health

g. food components (such as fibers) that are not digested by the human body but are used as food by the GI bacteria to promote their growth and activity

h. a hormone secreted by cells in the stomach wall that targets the glands of the stomach and stimulates secretion of gastric acid

i. a hormone produced by cells in the duodenum wall that targets the pancreas and stimulates secretion of bicarbonate-rich pancreatic juice

j. a hormone produced by cells of the intestinal wall that targets the gallbladder and stimulates release of bile and slowing of GI motility

Sample Test Questions

Select the best answer for each question.

1. The process by which food is broken down into absorbable units is called:
   a. absorption.
   b. digestion.
   c. peristalsis.
   d. reflux.

2. The uptake of nutrients by the cells in the small intestine for transport is called:
   a. absorption.
   b. digestion.
   c. circulation.
   d. segmentation.

3. The flexible muscular tube that extends from the mouth through the esophagus, stomach, small intestine, large intestine, and rectum to the anus is called:
   a. the lumen.
   b. the gastrointestinal tract.
   c. the bolus.
   d. segmentation.

4. The process of digestion begins in the:
   a. mouth.
   b. stomach.
   c. esophagus.
   d. small intestine.

5. Which organ crushes food and mixes it with saliva?
   a. Stomach
   b. Mouth
   c. Teeth
   d. Pharynx

6. After a mouthful of food has been swallowed, it is called:
   a. a crypt.
   b. chyme.
   c. a bolus.
   d. stool.

7. To keep food from entering the lungs, the _____ closes off air passages.
   a. pharynx
   b. diaphragm
   c. esophageal sphincter
   d. epiglottis

8. The wavelike muscular contractions that propel food through the digestive tract are called:
   a. defecation.
   b. peristalsis.
   c. hydrolysis.
   d. denaturation.

9. Which sphincter muscle is situated between the stomach and the small intestine?
   a. Cardiac sphincter
   b. Pyloric sphincter
   c. Ileocecal valve
   d. Rectal sphincter

10. The partially digested food that enters the small intestine from the stomach is called:
    a. micelles.
    b. bile.
    c. chyme.
    d. feces.

11. An enzyme that hydrolyzes proteins is called:
    a. bile.
    b. a sphincter valve.
    c. pancreatic amylase.
    d. a protease.
    e. a secretory peptide.

12. The main function of bile is to:
    a. emulsify fats.
    b. stimulate the activity of protein digestive enzymes.
    c. neutralize the contents of the intestine.
    d. increase peristalsis.
    e. a, b, and c

13. Which nutrients are digested in the small intestine?
    a. Carbohydrate, fat, and protein
    b. Fat, water, and fiber
    c. Protein, vitamins, and fiber
    d. Water, fiber, and minerals

14. A narrow blind sac extending from the beginning of the colon is called the:
    a. epiglottis.
    b. anus.
    c. rectum.
    d. appendix.

15. A single villus is composed of hundreds of _____, each covered with _____.
    a. organisms; mucus
    b. villi; lymph
    c. enzymes; mucus
    d. cells; microvilli
    e. crypts; glands

16. A group of cells that secrete materials for special uses in the body is:
    a. a gland.
    b. a sphincter.
    c. an enzyme.
    d. a hormone.

17. Avoiding certain food combinations at the same meal is:
    a. wise because the body cannot handle more than one task at a time.
    b. foolish because the body is equipped to handle digestion of a variety of foods and food types.
    c. practical and easy to adhere to.
    d. a and c

18. A periodic squeezing or partitioning of the intestines is:
    a. peristalsis.
    b. diverticulosis.
    c. segmentation.
    d. defecation.

19. The small intestine is about _____ feet long.
    a. 10
    b. 30
    c. 50
    d. 100

20. _____ muscles open and close, allowing the GI tract contents to move along at a controlled pace.
    a. Peristalsis
    b. Reflux
    c. Sphincter
    d. Segmentation

21. Glands that secrete intestinal juices into the small intestine are called:
    a. capillaries.
    b. microvilli.
    c. villi.
    d. crypts.

22. The strength of acids is measured in:
    a. ion concentrations.
    b. alkaline tests.
    c. base assessments.
    d. pH units.

23. Living microorganisms found in foods that benefit health are called:
    a. yogurt.
    b. probiotics.
    c. antibiotics.
    d. prebiotics.

24. Waste matter discharged from the colon is:
    a. a bolus.
    b. chyme.
    c. lymph.
    d. stools.

25. Saliva contains:
    a. proteases, bicarbonate, and water.
    b. bile, HCl, and water.
    c. chyme, pepsin, and bicarbonate.
    d. salts, carbohydrases, and water.
    e. a and b

26. The lymphatic system:
    a. contains red blood cells.
    b. eventually drains into the blood circulatory system.
    c. collects in a large duct behind the heart.
    d. a and b
    e. b and c

27. Which type of cells produce mucus that protects the stomach walls from gastric juices?
    a. Secretin
    b. Bile
    c. Cholecystokinin
    d. Goblet
    e. Enterogastrone

28. What hormone is released in the presence of fat and slows intestinal motility to allow a longer digestion time?
    a. Secretin
    b. Bile
    c. Cholecystokinin
    d. Gastrin
    e. Enterogastrone

29. The greatest danger from prolonged vomiting is:
    a. exhaustion.
    b. excess loss of fluid and salts.
    c. vitamin deficiencies.
    d. starvation.

30. A sensible idea for preventing constipation is to:
    a. take medication on a regular basis.
    b. cut down on water intake.
    c. include more high-fiber foods in the diet.
    d. include fewer high-fiber foods in the diet.

Short Answer Questions

1. Some problems involved in digestion include:

    a.

    b.

    c.

    d.

    e.

    f.

    g.

2. Organs and sphincters that foods pass through as they move through the digestive system include:

    a.   g.

    b.   h.

    c.   i.

    d.   j.

    e.   k.

    f.

3. Three processes by which nutrients are absorbed into the intestinal cells are:

    a.   c.

    b.

4. Three important structural features of the small intestine are:

    a.   c.

    b.

5. Three key structures of the blood circulatory system are:

    a.   c.

    b.

6. The nutrients that enter the lymphatic system prior to the bloodstream are:

    a.   b.

36

7. The potential GI health benefits of probiotics include:

a.

b.

c.

d.

e.

f.

g.

h.

i.

8. Three important (and extensively studied) GI hormones are:

a.

b.

c.

Figure Identification/Table Completion

A. **Identify the parts of the GI tract.**

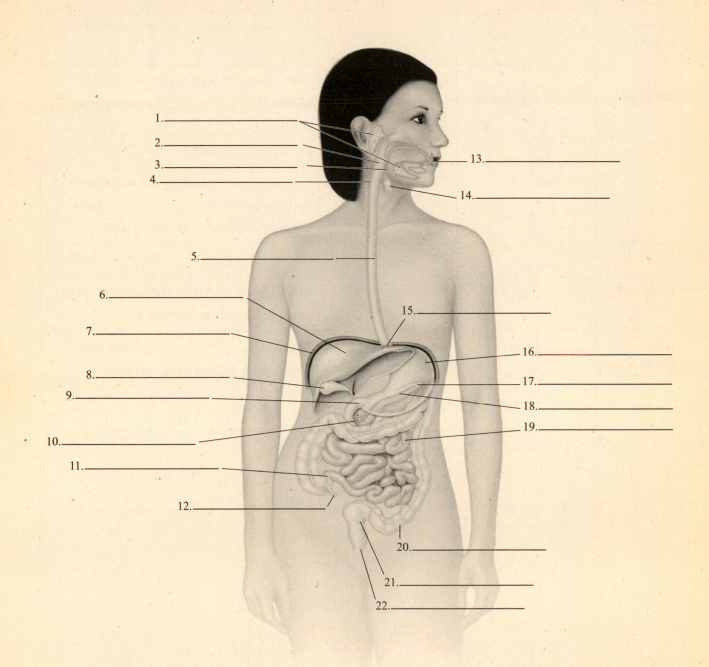

1. _____
2. _____
3. _____
4. _____
5. _____
6. _____
7. _____
8. _____
9. _____
10. _____
11. _____
12. _____
13. _____
14. _____
15. _____
16. _____
17. _____
18. _____
19. _____
20. _____
21. _____
22. _____

B. Complete this chart identifying digestive secretions and their primary actions.

Organ or Gland	Target Organ	Secretion	Action
Salivary glands	Mouth	1._____	Fluid eases swallowing; salivary enzyme breaks down some 2._____.
Gastric glands	3._____	Gastric juice	Fluid mixes with bolus; hydrochloric acid uncoils 4._____; enzymes break down 5._____; 6._____ protects stomach cells.
Pancreas	Small intestine	7._____	8._____ neutralizes acidic gastric juices; pancreatic 9._____ break down carbohydrates, fats, and proteins.
Liver	10._____	Bile	Bile stored until needed.
Gallbladder	11._____	Bile	Bile 12._____ fat so that enzymes can have access to break it down.
Intestinal glands	Small intestine	Intestinal juice	Intestinal 13._____ break down carbohydrate, fat, and protein fragments; 14._____ protects the intestinal wall.

C. **Complete the chart summarizing the chemical digestion and absorption that occur in each part of the GI tract.**

	Mouth	Stomach	Small Intestine	Large Intestine
Carbohydrate				
Fiber				
Protein				
Fat				
Vitamins				
Minerals				

❧ Chapter 3 Answer Key ❧

Summing Up

1. esophagus	9. salivary	17. lymph	25. hormonal
2. sphincters	10. pancreas	18. digestive	26. absorption
3. pyloric	11. gallbladder	19. liver	27. nutrients
4. ileocecal	12. digestive	20. cells	28. balanced
5. large intestine	13. villi	21. lymphatic	29. physical
6. rectum	14. surface	22. bypass	
7. peristalsis	15. absorption	23. bacteria	
8. segmentation	16. blood	24. GI	

Chapter Study Questions

1. The epiglottis closes off the airways so that food and liquid do not enter the lungs. Food passes through the diaphragm to reach the stomach by way of the esophagus. Fluids are added to the food as it travels through the system, allowing smooth passage. Water is reabsorbed in the large intestine (colon), thus conserving water and creating a semisolid waste. Peristalsis keeps the materials steadily moving through the system and sphincter muscles serve as one-way gates, allowing small quantities to pass at appropriate intervals. Stomach cells secrete mucus to protect them from acid and enzymes that would digest them. Rectal muscles prevent elimination until voluntarily performed.

2. Food enters the mouth and travels past the epiglottis, down the esophagus and through the lower esophageal (cardiac) sphincter to the stomach, then through the pyloric sphincter to the small intestine, on through the ileocecal valve to the large intestine, past the appendix to the rectum, ending at the anus. Muscular actions include: chewing, swallowing, peristalsis, segmentation, and sphincter contractions.

3. Salivary glands, stomach glands, pancreas, liver, gallbladder, and intestinal glands. Salivary glands secrete saliva, which contains amylase, an enzyme that breaks down starch. Gastric juice is secreted by the cells in the stomach wall and contains pepsin and HCl that break down proteins. Pancreatic juice contains bicarbonate that neutralizes acidic gastric juices as well as other enzymes that break down CHO, protein, and fat. The gallbladder secretes bile, which emulsifies fat.

4. The body must find a way to absorb many molecules. It solves this by its anatomy—the small intestine has hundreds of folds, each covered with thousands of villi, which in turn are composed of hundreds of cells, which in turn are covered with microvilli, providing a very large surface area for nutrient molecules to make contact and be absorbed.

5. Absorption of nutrients into intestinal cells occurs by simple diffusion, facilitated diffusion, or active transport. Water and small lipids are absorbed by simple diffusion (they cross into intestinal cells freely). The water-soluble vitamins are absorbed by facilitated diffusion. They need a specific carrier to transport them from one side of the cell membrane to the other. Glucose and amino acids must be absorbed actively. These nutrients move against a concentration gradient, which requires energy.

6. Heart to arteries to capillaries (in intestines) to vein (hepatic portal vein to the liver) to capillaries (in liver) to vein (hepatic vein) to heart. Water-soluble nutrients and small products of fat digestion enter the bloodstream directly; large fats and fat-soluble nutrients are first absorbed into the lymph.

7. The body's hormonal system and nervous system coordinate all the digestive and absorptive processes. The contents in the GI tract either stimulate or inhibit digestive secretions by way of messages that are carried from one section of the GI tract to another by both hormones and nerve pathways. For example, Food entering the stomach stimulates cells in the stomach wall to release the hormone gastrin, which stimulates the stomach glands to secrete the components of hydrochloric acid. Nerve receptors in the stomach wall also respond to the presence of food and stimulate the gastric glands to secrete juices and the muscles to contract. Likewise, fat in the intestine stimulates cells of the intestinal wall to release the hormone cholecystokinin (CCK), which stimulates the gallbladder to contract and release bile into the small intestine. Cholecystokinin also stimulates the pancreas to secrete bicarbonate and enzymes into the small intestine.

8. Four hundred or more different bacteria are present in a healthy GI tract. Most bacteria are not harmful but are health enhancing. A diverse and abundant bacteria population supports GI health. When the normal intestinal flora thrive, this makes it difficult for infectious bacteria to become established. The potential GI benefits of probiotics (live bacterial cultures found in yogurt) include helping to alleviate diarrhea, constipation, inflammatory bowel disease, ulcers, allergies, lactose intolerance, and infant colic. They may enhance immune function and protect against colon cancer.

9. Enzyme activity changes proportionately in response to the amounts of carbohydrate, fat, and protein in the diet. Hormones in the GI tract inform the pancreas as to the amount and type of enzymes to secrete in response to diet. The presence of fat slows GI motility.

10. Obtain adequate sleep, engage in physical activity, keep a positive state of mind, and eat meals with these characteristics: balance, moderation, variety, and adequacy.

Key Terms Practice

1. reflux	8. bolus	16. j	24. b
2. pH	9. crypts	17. g	25. g
3. A: chyme;	10. b	18. e	26. f
D: catalyst	11. a	19. f	27. i
4. flora	12. i	20. j	28. e
5. villi	13. d	21. h	29. d
6. stools	14. c	22. a	
7. yogurt	15. h	23. c	

Sample Test Questions

1. b (p. 69)	9. b (p. 73)	17. b (p. 79)	25. d (p. 74)
2. a (p. 69)	10. c (p. 72)	18. c (p. 73)	26. e (p. 82)
3. b (p. 70)	11. d (p. 74)	19. a (p. 77)	27. d (pp. 74-75, 78)
4. a (p. 71)	12. a (pp. 74, 75)	20. c (p. 73)	28. c (pp. 84, 85)
5. b (p. 71)	13. a (p. 75)	21. d (p. 78)	29. b (p. 90)
6. c (p. 72)	14. d (p. 72)	22. d (p. 75)	30. c (p. 91)
7. d (p. 72)	15. d (p. 78)	23. b (p. 83)	
8. b (p. 73)	16. a (p. 74)	24. d (p. 75)	

Short Answer Questions

1. a. Air and food must both come in through the mouth, but food and liquid must go to the stomach while air (but not food/liquid) goes into the lungs.
    b. Food must be conducted through the diaphragm to reach the abdomen.
    c. The materials within the tract should move steadily so that all reactions are completed.
    d. The amount of water should be regulated to keep the intestinal contents at the right consistency.
    e. Water must be withdrawn from the intestinal contents after absorption.
    f. The cells of the digestive tract need protection against the powerful juices they secrete.
    g. Provision must be made for periodic, voluntary evacuation when convenient.

2. mouth, upper esophageal sphincter, esophagus, lower esophageal sphincter, stomach, pyloric sphincter, small intestine, ileocecal valve, large intestine, rectum, anus

3. simple diffusion, facilitated diffusion, active transport

4. villi, microvilli, crypts

5. arteries, capillaries, veins

6. large fats, fat-soluble vitamins

7. helps to alleviate diarrhea, helps to alleviate constipation, helps to alleviate inflammatory bowel disease, helps to alleviate ulcers, helps to alleviate allergies, helps to alleviate lactose intolerance, helps to alleviate infant colic, may enhance immune function, may protect against colon cancer

8. gastrin, secretin, cholecystokinin

Figure Identification/Table Completion

A.
1. salivary glands
2. pharynx
3. epiglottis
4. upper esophageal sphincter
5. esophagus
6. liver
7. diaphragm
8. gallbladder
9. pyloric sphincter
10. bile duct
11. ileocecal valve
12. appendix
13. mouth
14. trachea
15. lower esophageal sphincter
16. stomach
17. pancreas
18. pancreatic duct
19. small intestine
20. large intestine
21. rectum
22. anus

B.
1. Saliva
2. carbohydrate
3. Stomach
4. proteins
5. proteins
6. mucus
7. Pancreatic juice
8. Bicarbonate
9. enzymes
10. Gallbladder
11. Small intestine
12. emulsifies
13. enzymes
14. mucus

C.

	Mouth	Stomach	Small Intestine	Large Intestine
Carbohydrate	Salivary enzyme begins to break down starch.	Digestion continues until HCl inactivates the salivary enzyme, then stops.	Sugars are absorbed. Pancreatic enzymes resume starch digestion. Intestinal cell enzymes complete starch digestion, and the resulting small fragments are absorbed into the hepatic portal vein.	None.
Fiber	None.	None.	None.	Some fibers are partially digested by bacteria; some of the products are absorbed. Most fibers are simply excreted.
Protein	None.	Begin to uncoil when mixed with gastric acid. Then gastric protease enzymes begin digestion.	Pancreatic and intestinal proteases complete digestion, and resulting small fragments are absorbed into the hepatic portal vein.	None.
Fat	Minimal in adults.	None.	Bile emulsifies fat. Pancreatic and intestinal lipases then digest it into small fragments that are absorbed into the lymph.	No digestion or absorption occur. Some fat and cholesterol bind to fiber and are excreted.
Vitamins	None.	None	Vitamins are absorbed.	None.
Minerals	None.	None	Minerals are absorbed.	Some minerals are absorbed; others bind to fiber and are excreted.

Chapter 4 ~ The Carbohydrates: Sugars, Starches, and Fibers

Chapter Outline

I. The Chemist's View of Carbohydrates
   A. Monosaccharides
      1. Glucose
      2. Fructose
      3. Galactose
   B. Disaccharides
      1. Condensation
      2. Hydrolysis
      3. Maltose
      4. Sucrose
      5. Lactose
   C. Polysaccharides
      1. Glycogen
      2. Starches
      3. Fibers
II. Digestion and Absorption of Carbohydrates
   A. Carbohydrate Digestion
      1. In the Mouth
      2. In the Stomach
      3. In the Small Intestine
      4. In the Large Intestine
   B. Carbohydrate Absorption
   C. Lactose Intolerance
      1. Symptoms
      2. Causes
      3. Prevalence
      4. Dietary Changes
III. Glucose in the Body
   A. A Preview of Carbohydrate Metabolism
      1. Storing Glucose as Glycogen
      2. Using Glucose for Energy
      3. Making Glucose from Protein
      4. Making Ketone Bodies from Fat Fragments
      5. Using Glucose to Make Fat
   B. The Constancy of Blood Glucose
      1. Maintaining Glucose Homeostasis
      2. The Regulating Hormones
      3. Balancing within the Normal Range
      4. Falling Outside the Normal Range
      5. Diabetes

6. Hypoglycemia
      7. The Glycemic Response
IV. Health Effects and Recommended Intakes of Sugars
   A. Health Effects of Sugars
      1. Obesity and Chronic Disease
      2. Nutrient Deficiencies
      3. Dental Caries
   B. Recommended Intakes of Sugars
   C. Alternative Sweeteners
      1. Artificial Sweeteners
      2. Stevia—An Herbal Sweetener
      3. Sugar Alcohols
V. Health Effects and Recommended Intakes of Starch and Fibers
   A. Health Effects of Starch and Fibers
      1. Heart Disease
      2. Diabetes
      3. GI Health
      4. Cancer
      5. Weight Management
      6. Harmful Effects of Excessive Fiber Intake
   B. Recommended Intakes of Starch and Fibers
   C. From Guidelines to Groceries
      1. Grains
      2. Vegetables
      3. Fruits
      4. Milks and Milk Products
      5. Protein Foods
      6. Read Food Labels
VI. Carbs, kCalories, and Controversies
   A. Carbohydrates' kCalorie Contributions
   B. Sugars' Share in the Problem
      1. Cravings and Addictions
      2. Appetite Control
   C. Insulin's Response
      1. The Glycemic Index and Body Weight
      2. The Individual's Response to Food
   D. In Summary

Summing Up

The carbohydrates are made of carbon, 1._____, and hydrogen. Each of these 2._____ can form a specified number of chemical bonds: 3._____ forms four, oxygen forms two, and hydrogen forms one.

The three monosaccharides (glucose, 4._____, and galactose) all have the same chemical formula ($C_6H_{12}O_6$), but their 5._____ differ. The three disaccharides (maltose, sucrose, and

44

6._____) are pairs of monosaccharides, each containing a 7._____ paired with one of the three monosaccharides. The sugars derive primarily from 8._____, except for lactose and its component galactose, which come from 9._____ and milk products. Two monosaccharides can be linked together by a 10._____ reaction to form a disaccharide and water. A disaccharide, in turn, can be broken into its two monosaccharides by a 11._____ reaction using water.

The 12._____ are chains of monosaccharides and include glycogen, starches, and dietary fibers. Both 13._____ and starch are storage forms of glucose—glycogen in the body, and starch in plants—and both yield 14._____ for human use. The dietary fibers also contain glucose (and other monosaccharides), but their bonds cannot be broken by 15._____ digestive enzymes, so they yield little, if any, energy.

In the digestion and absorption of carbohydrates, the body breaks down starches into the disaccharide 16._____. Maltose and the other disaccharides (lactose and sucrose) from foods are broken down into 17._____, which are absorbed. The 18._____ help to regulate the passage of food through the GI system and slow the absorption of glucose, but they contribute little, if any, 19._____.

Lactose intolerance is a common condition that occurs when there is insufficient 20._____ to digest the disaccharide lactose found in milk and milk products. Symptoms are limited to GI 21._____. Because treatment requires limiting milk and milk products in the diet, other sources of riboflavin, vitamin D, and calcium must be included.

Dietary carbohydrates provide glucose that can be used by the 22._____ for energy, stored by the liver and muscles as 23._____, or converted into fat if intakes exceed needs. All of the body's cells depend on 24._____; those of the central nervous system are especially dependent on it. Without glucose, the body is forced to break down its 25._____ tissues to make glucose and to alter energy metabolism to make 26._____ bodies from fats. Blood glucose regulation depends primarily on two pancreatic hormones: 27._____ to move glucose from the blood into the cells when levels are high and 28._____ to free glucose from glycogen stores and release it into the blood when levels are low.

Sugars increase the risk of 29._____ caries; excessive intakes displace needed nutrients and fiber and contribute to 30._____ when energy intake exceeds needs. A person deciding to limit daily sugar intake should recognize that not all sugars need to be restricted, just 31._____ sweets, which are relatively 32._____ of other nutrients and high in kcalories. Sugars that occur naturally in fruits, vegetables, and milk are 33._____. Alternative 34._____ may help to limit kcalories and sugar intake.

Clearly, a diet rich in starches and 35._____ supports efforts to control body weight and prevent heart disease, some 36._____, diabetes, and GI disorders. For these reasons, recommendations urge people to eat plenty of whole grains, vegetables, 37._____, and fruits—enough to provide 45 to 65 percent of the daily energy intake from carbohydrate.

Chapter Study Questions

1. Which carbohydrates are described as simple and which are complex?

2. Describe the structure of a monosaccharide and name the three monosaccharides important in nutrition. Name the three disaccharides commonly found in foods and their component monosaccharides. In what foods are these sugars found?

3. What happens in a condensation reaction? In a hydrolysis reaction?

4. Describe the structure of polysaccharides and name the ones important in nutrition. How are starch and glycogen similar and how do they differ? How do the fibers differ from the other polysaccharides?

5. Describe carbohydrate digestion and absorption. What role does fiber play in the process?

6. What is lactose intolerance and how can a person with lactose intolerance manage the condition while maintaining nutrient adequacy?

46

7. What are the possible fates of glucose in the body? What is the protein-sparing action of carbohydrate?

8. How does the body maintain blood glucose concentrations? What happens when blood glucose rises too high or falls too low?

9. What are the health effects of sugars? What are the dietary recommendations regarding concentrated sugar intakes?

10. What are the three major categories of alternative sweeteners? What are the recommendations regarding the use of these sweeteners?

11. What are the health effects of starches and fibers? What are the dietary recommendations regarding these complex carbohydrates?

12. What foods provide starches and fibers?

Key Terms Practice

To complete the crossword puzzle, identify the key term that best matches each definition.

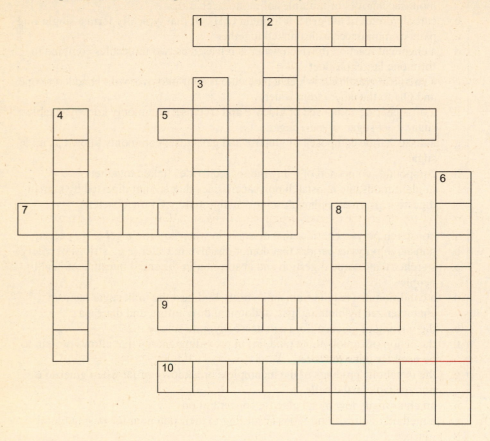

Across:
1. Simple carbohydrates composed of monosaccharides or disaccharides.
5. A hormone that is secreted by special cells in the pancreas in response to low blood glucose concentration and elicits release of glucose from liver glycogen stores.
7. A monosaccharide that is sometimes known as fruit sugar or levulose.
9. A hormone secreted by special cells in the pancreas in response to (among other things) increased blood glucose concentration.
10. A monosaccharide; part of the disaccharide lactose.

Down:
2. A monosaccharide that is sometimes known as blood sugar in the body or dextrose in foods.
3. An animal polysaccharide composed of glucose; it is manufactured and stored in the liver and muscles as a storage form of glucose.
4. Plant polysaccharides composed of many glucose units.
6. A chronic disorder of carbohydrate metabolism, usually resulting from insufficient or ineffective insulin.
8. The feeling of fullness and satisfaction that occurs after a meal and inhibits eating until the next meal.

Match the key terms with their definitions.

11. _____ carbohydrates

12. _____ condensation

13. _____ dietary fibers

14. _____ disaccharides

15. _____ hydrolysis

16. _____ lactose

17. _____ monosaccharides

18. _____ polysaccharides

19. _____ sucrose

a. compounds composed of carbon, oxygen, and hydrogen arranged as monosaccharides or multiples of monosaccharides

b. carbohydrates of the general formula $C_nH_{2n}O_n$ that typically form a single ring

c. pairs of monosaccharides linked together

d. a chemical reaction in which water is released as two molecules combine to form one larger product

e. a chemical reaction in which a molecule is split into two, with H added to one and OH to the other (from water)

f. a disaccharide composed of glucose and fructose; commonly known as table sugar, beet sugar, or cane sugar

g. a disaccharide composed of glucose and galactose; commonly known as milk sugar

h. compounds composed of many monosaccharides linked together

i. in plant foods, the nonstarch polysaccharides that are not digested by human digestive enzymes, although some are digested by GI tract bacteria

20. _____ artificial sweeteners

21. _____ dental caries

22. _____ gluconeogenesis

23. _____ glycemic index

24. _____ hypoglycemia

25. _____ insoluble fibers

26. _____ ketone bodies

27. _____ lactose intolerance

28. _____ protein-sparing action

29. _____ resistant starches

30. _____ soluble fibers

a. nonstarch polysaccharides that dissolve in water to form a gel (e.g., pectin)

b. nonstarch polysaccharides that do not dissolve in water (e.g., strings of celery)

c. starches that escape digestion and absorption in the small intestine of healthy people

d. a condition that results from an inability to digest the milk sugar lactose; characterized by bloating, gas, abdominal discomfort, and diarrhea

e. the making of glucose from a noncarbohydrate source

f. the action of carbohydrate (and fat) in providing energy that allows protein to be used for other purposes

g. the metabolic products of the incomplete breakdown of fat when glucose is not available in the cells

h. an abnormally low blood glucose concentration

i. a method of classifying foods according to their potential for raising blood glucose

j. decay of teeth

k. sugar substitutes that provide negligible, if any, energy

Sample Test Questions

Select the best answer for each question.

1. Carbohydrates appear in virtually all _____ foods.
   a. plant
   b. animal
   c. high-fat
   d. protein

2. Carbohydrates are made of the following 3 atoms:
   a. carbon, oxygen, and nitrogen.
   b. carbon, oxygen, and hydrogen.
   c. nitrogen, oxygen, and hydrogen.
   d. cadmium, oxygen, and hydrogen.

3. Which of the following compounds is a monosaccharide?
   a. Sucrose
   b. Fructose
   c. Maltose
   d. Lactose
   e. Pectin

4. Which of the following are disaccharides?
   a. Glucose, maltose
   b. Fructose, sucrose
   c. Galactose, lactose
   d. Maltose, sucrose

5. Fructose is the sweetest of sugars because:
   a. its chemical structure stimulates a sweet sensation.
   b. its chemical formula resembles glucose.
   c. it provides more kcalories than other sugars.
   d. it occurs naturally in honey.

6. A hydrolysis reaction can:
   a. bond two monosaccharides to form a disaccharide.
   b. split a disaccharide to form two monosaccharides.
   c. form a molecule of water.
   d. a and c
   e. b and c

7. What type of reaction links two monosaccharides together?
   a. Disaccharide
   b. Hydrolysis
   c. Absorption
   d. Condensation

8. Disaccharides include:
   a. glucose.
   b. maltose.
   c. glycogen.
   d. sucrose.
   e. b and d

9. The principal carbohydrate of milk is:
   a. lactose.
   b. sucrose.
   c. maltose.
   d. glycogen.

10. Fruits are usually sweet because they contain:
    a. fiber.
    b. complex carbohydrates.
    c. simple sugars.
    d. fats.

11. An animal polysaccharide composed of glucose is called:
    a. fiber.
    b. dextrins.
    c. glycogen.
    d. starch.

12. The difference between glycogen and starch is:
    a. the bonds in starch are fatty acids.
    b. the bonds in starch are single.
    c. the bonds in glycogen are not hydrolyzed by human enzymes.
    d. the glucose units are arranged differently.

13. Starch is made up of many glucose units bonded together.
    a. True
    b. False

14. Fibers that do not dissolve in water are:
    a. soluble fibers.
    b. viscous fibers.
    c. fermentable fibers.
    d. insoluble fibers.

15. Which type of starches escapes digestion and absorption in the small intestine?
    a. Functional starches
    b. Phytic starches
    c. Resistant starches
    d. Plant starches

16. Most carbohydrate absorption occurs in the:
    a.   mouth.
    b.   stomach.
    c.   small intestine.
    d.   large intestine.
    e.   b and c

17. An enzyme that hydrolyzes sucrose is:
    a.   glucose.
    b.   lactase.
    c.   pectin.
    d.   sucrase.

18. Carbohydrate digestion occurs in:
    a.   the stomach and small intestine.
    b.   the mouth and small intestine.
    c.   the stomach and colon.
    d.   the mouth and pancreas.

19. A condition that results from an inability to digest lactose is called:
    a.   lactose deficiency.
    b.   lactose intolerance.
    c.   hypoglycemia.
    d.   lactase intolerance.

20. The main function of carbohydrate in the body is to:
    a.   furnish the body with energy.
    b.   provide materials for synthesizing cell walls.
    c.   synthesize fat.
    d.   insulate the body to prevent heat loss.

21. When blood glucose levels fall, the liver:
    a.   combines excess glucose molecules.
    b.   stores glucose as glycogen.
    c.   dismantles stored glycogen.
    d.   combines glucose to form molecules of fat.

22. The conversion of protein to glucose is called:
    a.   ketosis.
    b.   protein-sparing action.
    c.   glycogenolysis.
    d.   gluconeogenesis.

23. Which of the following is true regarding ketosis?
    a.   It is a desirable state for weight maintenance.
    b.   It is a condition that disturbs the body's acid-base balance.
    c.   It occurs when people eat too many kcalories.
    d.   It results from the body's breakdown of protein.

24. What hormone signals the release of glucose out of storage?
    a.   Glucagon
    b.   Insulin
    c.   Testosterone
    d.   Secretin

25. What condition results in the body's cells failing to respond to insulin?
    a.   Hyperlipidemia
    b.   Hypoglycemia
    c.   Type 1 diabetes
    d.   Type 2 diabetes

26. _____ refers to how quickly glucose is absorbed after a person eats and how high blood sugar rises.
    a.   Hypoglycemia
    b.   Hyperglycemia
    c.   Glycemic response
    d.   Glycemic load

27. Sugar causes:
    a.   addictions.
    b.   diabetes.
    c.   ulcers.
    d.   dental caries.
    e.   All of the above

28. Taken with ample fluids, fibers can help prevent:
    a. hemorrhoids.
    b. appendicitis.
    c. hyperactivity.
    d. a and b
    e. b and c

29. Dietary fiber:
    a. raises blood cholesterol levels.
    b. is found in high-fat foods.
    c. causes diverticulosis.
    d. provides satiety and delays hunger.

30. Excess fiber can result in:
    a. abdominal discomfort.
    b. gas and diarrhea.
    c. dental caries.
    d. a and b
    e. a, b, and c

31. Which of the following is true regarding alternative sweeteners?
    a. They are harmful and should not be used.
    b. They may help prevent dental caries.
    c. They should be used in place of all sugars.
    d. They may help control weight gain and blood glucose.
    e. b and d
    f. c and d

Short Answer Questions

1. Hormones involved in maintaining blood glucose are:

    a.   c.

    b.

2. The monosaccharides are:

    a.   c.

    b.

3. The disaccharides are:

    a.   c.

    b.

4. The polysaccharides are:

    a.   c.

    b.

5. The enzymes that break down disaccharides are:

    a.   c.

    b.

6. Symptoms of lactose intolerance include:

    a.   c.

    b.   d.

52

7. Three ways carbohydrate can be used in the body are:

a.   c.

b.

8. The names and descriptions of the two primary types of diabetes are:

a.

b.

9. Steps people can take to limit dental caries include:

a.

b.

c.

d.

e.

10. The three types of alternative sweeteners are:

a.   c.

b.

11. Diseases that may be prevented or managed through healthy intakes of carbohydrates and fiber include:

a.   d.

b.   e.

c.

12. Four harmful effects of consuming excessive fiber are:

a.   c.

b.   d.

Problem Solving

1. About how many grams of carbohydrate are in the following meal?
   2 slices whole-wheat bread with
   1 oz. cheddar cheese
   1 pat butter
   1 small orange

2. Based on this estimate, about how many kcalories do carbohydrates contribute to the meal above?

3. The meal provides 365 kcalories. What percentage of the kcalories is from carbohydrates?

4. For a person whose energy requirement is 1500 kcalories per day, calculate the number of grams of carbohydrate necessary to provide 55% of kcalories from carbohydrate.

5. For a person whose energy requirement is 2500 kcalories per day, calculate the number of grams of carbohydrate necessary to provide 55% of kcalories from carbohydrate.

6. If a person consumed 31 teaspoons of white sugar, how many kcalories did they ingest?

7. A person who consumes 10 oz. of regular carbonated soda is taking in how many kcalories?

8. A person whose energy needs are 2000 kcalories per day consumes 10 tablespoons of ketchup. How many kcalories were provided by the ketchup, and what percentage of total daily kcalories came from the ketchup alone?

9. If you consume 1.5 cups of dry oat bran, how many grams of fiber does this provide?

10. If a label indicates that a product provides 20 g of total carbohydrate, 2 grams of dietary fiber, and 5 grams of sugar, how many grams of starch does it provide?

Figure Identification

Identify these structures and reactions.

1.

2.

3.

4.

CH$_2$OH CH$_2$OH   CH$_2$OH CH$_2$OH

HO OH   OH   H—O OH   OH   HO OH   OH   OH

OH   OH   OH   OH

$\longrightarrow$

                                  +

H$_2$O   H$_2$O
Water   Water

5.

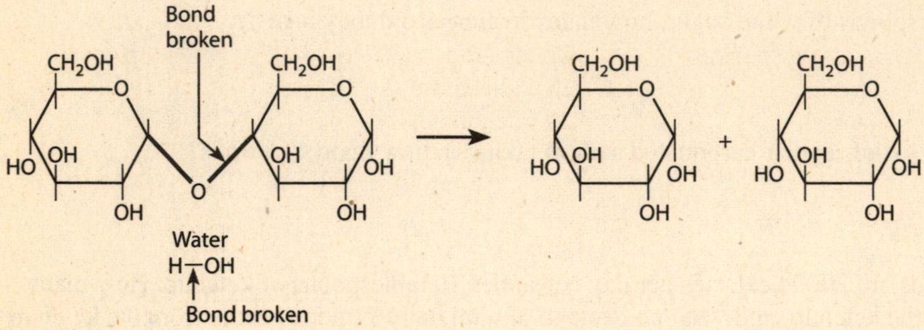

Bond
broken

CH$_2$OH   CH$_2$OH   CH$_2$OH   CH$_2$OH

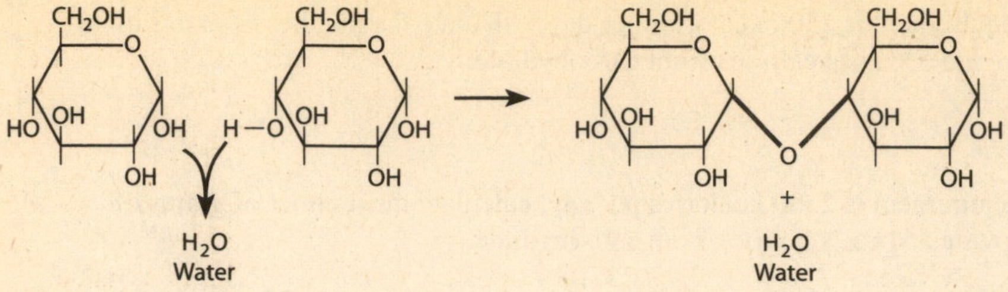

HO OH   OH   OH   HO OH   OH   HO OH   OH

OH   OH   OH   OH

$\longrightarrow$ +

O

Water
H—OH

Bond broken

6.

❧ Chapter 4 Answer Key ❧

Summing Up

1. oxygen	11. hydrolysis	21. distress	31. concentrated
2. atoms	12. polysaccharides	22. cells	32. empty
3. carbon	13. glycogen	23. glycogen	33. acceptable
4. fructose	14. energy	24. glucose	34. sweeteners
5. structures	15. human	25. protein	35. fibers
6. lactose	16. maltose	26. ketone	36. cancers
7. glucose	17. monosaccharides	27. insulin	37. legumes
8. plants	18. fibers	28. glucagon	
9. milk	19. energy	29. dental	
10. condensation	20. lactase	30. obesity	

Chapter Study Questions

1   Simple—monosaccharides (glucose, fructose, galactose), disaccharides (sucrose, lactose, maltose). Complex—glycogen and starch.

2. A monosaccharide is a carbohydrate, usually with a single-ring structure, that is composed of carbon, hydrogen, and oxygen atoms (general formula $C_nH_{2n}O_n$). Monosaccharides important in nutrition are glucose, fructose, and galactose; disaccharides important in nutrition are sucrose (fructose + glucose), lactose (galactose + glucose), and maltose (2 glucoses). Nearly all plant foods contain glucose, and most plants (especially fruits and saps) contain fructose. Galactose is rarely found as such in foods. Sucrose occurs in many fruits and some vegetables and grains. Lactose is found in milk, and maltose is found in seeds.

3. Condensation combines two reactants to yield one product with the release of water; hydrolysis splits one reactant into two products with the addition of water.

4. Polysaccharides are composed of many monosaccharides strung together. Important in nutrition are: glycogen, starch, and the fibers. Starch and glycogen are similar in that they are both composed of glucose; they differ in the way their glucose units are arranged. Glycogen consists of many glucose molecules linked together in highly branched chains, while starch consists of many glucose molecules linked in long, branched or straight chains. Fibers are different in that the bonds between their monosaccharides cannot be broken by human enzymes.

5. Salivary amylase enzymes in the mouth partially break down some of the starch before it reaches the intestine, pancreatic enzymes digest the starch to disaccharides in the small intestine, and disaccharidase enzymes on surface of intestinal wall cells split disaccharides to monosaccharides. Monosaccharides enter the circulatory system via a capillary. The blood delivers monosaccharides to the liver, and the liver converts galactose and fructose to compounds within the same metabolic pathways as glucose. Glucose is released by the liver for delivery by the blood to other body cells. In the mouth, fiber slows the process of eating and stimulates the flow of saliva; in the stomach, fiber delays gastric emptying; in the small intestine, it delays absorption of carbohydrates and fats, and can bind with minerals; in the large intestine, it attracts water that softens the stools.

6. Lactose intolerance results from an inability to digest the milk sugar lactose. It is characterized by bloating, gas, abdominal discomfort, and diarrhea. People with lactose intolerance may consider some dietary modifications but most need not exclude all milk products. They can increase consumption of lactose-containing products gradually, consume them with meals, and spread their intake throughout the day. Certain cheeses, including cheddar and cottage cheese, are well tolerated. Yogurt containing live bacteria seems to improve lactose intolerance. Most people with lactose intolerance need to manage dietary lactose rather than restrict it.

7. It can be stored as glycogen; it can be used for energy; it can be converted to fat. Glucose can be used for energy, leaving protein available for its special functions.

8. Hormones are secreted in response to fluctuations in blood glucose. When blood glucose is too high, the pancreas releases insulin, resulting in the storage of glucose in the cells; when blood glucose is too low, the pancreas releases glucagon, resulting in the release of glucose into the blood.

9. Excess sugar can cause malnutrition if sugar displaces needed nutrients from the diet. It can contribute to obesity. Excess sugar can contribute to elevated blood lipids, and it can cause dental caries. The *Dietary Guidelines for Americans* advise that kcal intake from added sugars be reduced. The DRI recommend that no more than 25% of kcal intake should come from added sugars, whereas the World Health Organization suggests they should not exceed 10% of kcal intake.

10. Alternative sweeteners are selected to help people limit kcalories and minimize sugar intake. The three categories are artificial sweeteners, an herbal sweetener (stevia), and sugar alcohols. Artificial sweeteners are sugar substitutes that provide negligible, if any, energy. Stevia is derived from a plant used as a sweetener by people in South America. Sugar alcohols are reduced-kcalorie products that are absorbed more slowly than other sugars and metabolized differently. They are not readily used by ordinary mouth bacteria. They do provide some kcalories and are considered nutritive sweeteners. Alternative sweeteners should be used in moderation and only as part of a well-balanced, nutritious diet.

11. They protect against heart disease, possibly colon cancer, and diabetes; assist in weight control; improve large intestinal function and health; lower blood cholesterol levels; and slow the rate of glucose absorption. Forty-five to 65% of total kcalories should come from carbohydrate: mostly from starch, some from fruits, vegetables, and milk. The RDA is 130 g/day. The Daily Value for carbohydrate is 300 g. The DRI recommendation for fiber is 14 g per 1000 kcalories, or about 25-35 g/day. The Daily Value recommendation for fiber is 25 grams of fiber (based on 11.5 g per 1000 kcalories).

12. Fruits (fresh, frozen, and dried fruits) provide variable amounts of fiber; fruit juices contain little fiber. Vegetables (cooked or raw vegetables including broccoli, cabbage, cauliflower, collards, spinach, squash, carrots, etc.), legumes (cooked baked beans, black beans, black-eyed peas, kidney beans, navy beans, pinto beans), and whole grains (whole-grain breads, cereals, other products) provide starches and fibers.

Key Terms Practice

1. sugars	9. insulin	17. b	25. b
2. glucose	10. galactose	18. h	26. g
3. glycogen	11. a	19. f	27. d
4. starches	12. d	20. k	28. f
5. glucagon	13. i	21. j	29. c
6. diabetes	14. c	22. e	30. a
7. fructose	15. e	23. i	
8. satiety	16. g	24. h	

Sample Test Questions

1. a (p. 95)	9. a (p. 99)	17. d (p. 101)	25. d (p. 107)
2. b (p. 95)	10. c (p. 97)	18. b (p. 101)	26. c (p. 108)
3. b (p. 96)	11. c (p. 99)	19. b (p. 103)	27. d (p. 111)
4. d (p. 96)	12. d (p. 99)	20. a (p. 106)	28. d (p. 116)
5. a (p. 97)	13. a (p. 99)	21. c (p. 105)	29. d (p. 117)
6. b (p. 98)	14. d (p. 100)	22. d (p. 105)	30. d (p. 117)
7. d (p. 98)	15. c (p. 100)	23. b (p. 106)	31. e (pp. 113-114)
8. e (pp. 96, 98)	16. c (p. 103)	24. a (p. 106)	

Short Answer Questions

1. insulin, glucagon, epinephrine

2. glucose, fructose, galactose

3. maltose, sucrose, lactose

4. starch, glycogen, fiber

5. maltase, sucrose, lactase

6. bloating, gas, abdominal discomfort, diarrhea

7. stored as glycogen; broken down to release energy; made into fat

8. type I diabetes—the pancreas fails to produce insulin; type 2 diabetes—cells fail to respond to the produced insulin

9. limit between-meal snacks; brush with fluoride toothpaste; floss daily; obtain dental check-ups regularly; drink fluoridated water

10. artificial sweeteners, herbal sweeteners (stevia), sugar alcohols

11. heart disease, diabetes, GI tract disorders, cancer, obesity/overweight

12. abdominal discomfort, gas, diarrhea, GI tract obstruction

Problem Solving

1. $2 (15 \text{ g}) + 0 + 0 + 15 \text{ g} = 45 \text{ g}$

2. $4 \text{ kcal/g} \times 45 \text{ g} = 180 \text{ kcal}$

3. 180 kcal divided by 365 kcal = 49%

4. $1500 \text{ kcal} \times 0.55 = 825 \text{ kcal}$ divided by 4 kcal/gram = 206 grams

5. $2500 \text{ kcal} \times 0.55 = 1375 \text{ kcal}$ divided by 4 kcal/gram = 344 grams

6. $31 \text{ teaspoons} \times 16 \text{ kcalories/teaspoon} = 496 \text{ kcalories}$

7. 1.5 oz = 20 kcalories
   20 divided by 1.5 = 13.3 kcalories per ounce
   $10 \text{ oz.} \times 13.3 \text{ kcal per oz.} = 133 \text{ kcalories}$

8. $10 \text{ tbsp} \times 20 \text{ kcalories} = 200 \text{ kcalories}$
   200 divided by 2000 = 10% of kcalorie needs

9. 0.5 cups = 8 grams fiber
   1.5 divided by 0.5 = 3
   $3 \times 8 = 24 \text{ grams}$

10. 20 g total − 2 grams dietary fiber − 5 grams sugar = 13 g starch

Figure Identification

1. glucose
2. glucose
3. fructose
4. galactose
5. condensation reaction
6. hydrolysis reaction

✆ Chapter 5 ~ The Lipids: ✆
Triglycerides, Phospholipids, and Sterols

Chapter Outline

I. The Chemist's View of Fatty Acids and Triglycerides
  A. Fatty Acids
    1. The Length of the Carbon Chain
    2. The Number of Double Bonds
    3. The Location of Double Bonds
  B. Triglycerides
  C. Characteristics of Solid Fats and Oils
    1. Firmness
    2. Stability
    3. Hydrogenation
    4. *Trans*-Fatty Acids
II. The Chemist's View of Phospholipids and Sterols
  A. Phospholipids
    1. Phospholipids in Foods
    2. Roles of Phospholipids
  B. Sterols
    1. Sterols in Foods
    2. Roles of Sterols
III. Digestion, Absorption, and Transport of Lipids
  A. Lipid Digestion
    1. In the Mouth
    2. In the Stomach
    3. In the Small Intestine
    4. Bile's Routes
  B. Lipid Absorption
  C. Lipid Transport
    1. Chylomicrons
    2. VLDL (Very-Low-Density Lipoproteins)
    3. LDL (Low-Density Lipoproteins)
    4. HDL (High-Density Lipoproteins)
    5. Health Implications
IV. Lipids in the Body
  A. Roles of Triglycerides
  B. Essential Fatty Acids
    1. Linoleic Acid and the Omega-6 Family
    2. Linolenic Acid and the Omega-3 Family
    3. Eicosanoids
    4. Omega-6 to Omega-3 Ratio

    5. Fatty Acid Deficiencies
  C. A Preview of Lipid Metabolism
    1. Storing Fat as Fat
    2. Using Fat for Energy
V. Health Effects and Recommended Intakes of Saturated Fats, *Trans* Fats, and Cholesterol
  A. Health Effects of Saturated Fats, *Trans* Fats, and Cholesterol
    1. Heart Disease
    2. Cancer
    3. Obesity
  B. Recommended Intakes of Saturated Fat, *Trans* Fat, and Cholesterol
VI. Health Effects and Recommended Intakes of Monounsaturated and Polyunsaturated Fats
  A. Health Effects of Monounsaturated and Polyunsaturated Fats
    1. Heart Disease
    2. Cancer
    3. Omega-3 Supplements
  B. Recommended Intakes of Monounsaturated and Polyunsaturated Fats
  C. From Guidelines to Groceries
    1. Protein Foods
    2. Milk and Milk Products
    3. Vegetables, Fruits, and Grains
    4. Solid Fats and Oils
    5. Read Food Labels
    6. Fat Replacers
VII. High-Fat Foods—Friend or Foe?
  A. Guidelines for Fat Intake
  B. High-Fat Foods and Heart Health
    1. Cook with Olive Oil
    2. Nibble on Nuts
    3. Feast on Fish
  C. High-Fat Foods and Heart Disease
    1. Limit Fatty Meats, Whole-Milk Products, and Tropical Oils
    2. Limit Hydrogenated Foods
  D. The Mediterranean Diet
  E. Conclusion

Summing Up

The predominant lipids both in foods and in the body are 1._____: a molecule of

2._____ with three fatty acids attached. Fatty acids vary in the length of their carbon chains, their

degrees of 3._____ (number of double bonds), and the 4._____ of their double bond(s). Those that are fully loaded with hydrogens are 5._____; those that are missing hydrogens and therefore have 6._____ are unsaturated (monounsaturated or 7._____). The vast majority of triglycerides contain more than one type of 8._____. Fatty acid saturation affects fats' physical characteristics and 9._____ properties. Hydrogenation, which converts polyunsaturated fats to 10._____ fats, protects fats from 11._____ and alters the texture by making liquid vegetable oils more 12._____. In the process, hydrogenation creates 13._____-fatty acids that 14._____ health in ways similar to those of saturated fatty acids.

Phospholipids, including lecithin, have a unique chemical structure that allows them to be 15._____ in both water and fat. The food industry uses phospholipids as 16._____, and in the body, phospholipids are part of cell 17._____. 18._____ have a multiple-ring structure that differs from the structure of other lipids. In the body, sterols include 19._____, bile, vitamin D, and some hormones. Animal-derived foods are rich sources of cholesterol.

The body makes special arrangements to digest and 20._____ lipids. It provides the emulsifier 21._____ to make them accessible to the fat-digesting lipases that dismantle triglycerides, mostly to 22._____ and fatty acids, for absorption by the intestinal cells. The intestinal cells assemble absorbed lipids into 23._____, lipid packages with protein escorts, for transport so that 24._____ all over the body may select needed lipids from them. Lipoproteins transport 25._____ around the body. All four types of 26._____ carry all classes of lipids (triglycerides, phospholipids, and cholesterol), but the 27._____ are the largest and contain mostly 28._____ from the diet; VLDL are smaller and are about 29._____ triglycerides; LDL are smaller still and contain mostly 30._____; and HDL are the densest and are rich in 31._____. High LDL cholesterol indicates increased risk of 32._____ disease, whereas high HDL cholesterol has a 33._____ effect.

In the body, triglycerides provide energy, insulate against temperature extremes, protect against shock, provide 34._____ material for cell membranes, and participate in cell signaling pathways. Linoleic acid (18 carbons, omega-6) and linolenic acid (18 carbons, omega-3) are 35._____ nutrients. They serve as structural parts of cell membranes and as precursors to the longer fatty acids that can make 36._____—powerful compounds that participate in blood pressure regulation, blood clot formation, and the 37._____ response to injury and infection, among other functions. Because essential fatty acids are common in the diet and stored in the body, 38._____ are unlikely. The body can easily store unlimited amounts of 39._____ if given excesses, and this body fat is used for energy when needed.

Although some fat in the diet is necessary, too much fat adds kcalories without 40._____, which leads to obesity and nutrient inadequacies. Too much saturated fat, *trans* fat, and cholesterol increase the risk of 41._____ disease and possibly cancer. For these reasons, health authorities recommend a diet moderate in total fat and 42._____ in saturated fat, *trans* fat, and cholesterol.

60

Some fat in the diet has health benefits, especially the 43._____ and

polyunsaturated fats that protect against heart disease and possibly 44._____. For this reason, the *Dietary*

Guidelines recommend replacing saturated fats with monounsaturated and polyunsaturated fats, particularly

45._____ fatty acids from foods such as fatty fish, not from supplements. Many selection and preparation

strategies can help bring these goals within reach, and 46._____ labels help to identify foods consistent with

these guidelines.

Chapter Study Questions

1. Name the three classes of lipids found in the body and in foods. What are some of their functions in the body? What features do fats bring to foods?

2. What features distinguish fatty acids from each other?

3. What does the term "omega" mean with respect to fatty acids? Describe omega-3 and omega-6 fatty acids.

4. What are the differences among saturated, unsaturated, monounsaturated, and polyunsaturated fats? Describe the structure of a triglyceride.

5. What does hydrogenation do to fat? What are *trans*-fatty acids, and how do they influence heart disease risk?

6. How do phospholipids differ from triglycerides in structure? How does cholesterol differ? How do these differences in structure affect function?

7. What roles do phospholipids play in the body? What roles does cholesterol play in the body?

8. Trace the steps in fat digestion, absorption, and transport. Describe the routes cholesterol takes in the body.

9. What do lipoproteins do? What are the differences among the chylomicrons, VLDL, LDL, and HDL?

10. Which of the fatty acids are essential? Name their chief dietary sources.

11. How does excessive fat intake influence health? What factors influence LDL, HDL, and total blood cholesterol?

12. What are the dietary recommendations regarding saturated fat, *trans* fat, and cholesterol intake?

13. Describe the relationship between monounsaturated and polyunsaturated fatty acids and health.

14. What is the Daily Value for fat? What does this number represent?

15. List recommendations for a heart-healthy diet.

Key Terms Practice

To complete the crossword puzzle, identify the key term that best matches each definition.

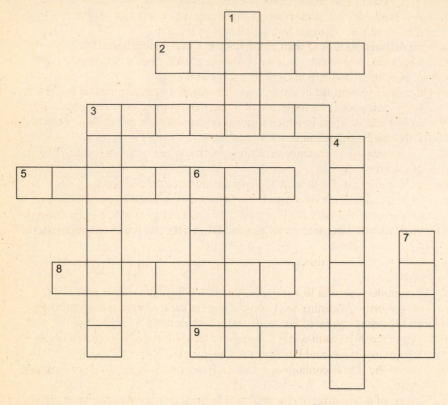

Across:

2. An accumulation of fatty deposits, smooth muscle cells, and fibrous connective tissue that develops in the artery walls in atherosclerosis.
3. Enzymes that hydrolyze lipids.
5. Tiny spherical complexes of emulsified fat that arise during digestion; most contain bile salts and the products of lipid digestion, including fatty acids, monoglycerides, and cholesterol.
8. A nitrogen-containing compound found in foods and made in the body from the amino acid methionine.
9. Compounds containing a four-ring carbon structure with any of a variety of side chains attached.

Down:

1. Lipids that are solid at room temperature (77°F or 25°C).
3. One of the phospholipids; it is used as an emulsifier to combine water-soluble and fat-soluble ingredients that do not ordinarily mix, such as water and oil.
4. An alcohol composed of a three-carbon chain, which can serve as the backbone for a triglyceride.
6. A family of compounds that includes triglycerides, phospholipids, and sterols.
7. Lipids that are liquid at room temperature (77°F or 25°C).

Match the key terms with their definitions.

10. _____ antioxidants

11. _____ condensation

12. _____ hydrogenation

13. _____ linoleic acid

14. _____ linolenic acid

15. _____ omega-3 fatty acid

16. _____ omega-6 fatty acid

17. _____ oxidation

18. _____ *trans*-fatty acids

19. _____ triglycerides

a. a polyunsaturated fatty acid in which the closest double bond to the methyl (CH_3) end of the carbon chain is three carbons away

b. as a food additive, preservatives that delay or prevent rancidity of fats in foods and other damage to food caused by oxygen

c. an essential fatty acid with 18 carbons and two double bonds

d. a polyunsaturated fatty acid in which the closest double bond to the methyl (CH_3) end of the carbon chain is six carbons away

e. the chief form of fat in the diet and the major storage form of fat in the body; composed of a molecule of glycerol with three fatty acids attached

f. a chemical reaction in which water is released as two molecules combine to form one larger product

g. the process of a substance combining with oxygen, which involves the loss of electrons

h. an essential fatty acid with 18 carbons and three double bonds

i. a chemical process by which hydrogens are added to monounsaturated or polyunsaturated fatty acids to reduce the number of double bonds, making the fats more saturated (solid) and more resistant to oxidation (protecting against rancidity)

j. fatty acids with hydrogens on opposite sides of the double bond

20. _____ adipose tissue

21. _____ atherosclerosis

22. _____ cholesterol

23. _____ chylomicrons

24. _____ emulsifiers

25. _____ essential fatty acids

26. _____ high-density lipoprotein

27. _____ lipoproteins

28. _____ monoglycerides

29. _____ phospholipid

a. a compound similar to a triglyceride but having a phosphate group (a phosphorus-containing salt) and choline (or another nitrogen-containing compound) in place of one of the fatty acids

b. substances with both water-soluble and fat-soluble portions that promote the mixing of oils and fats in watery solutions

c. one of the sterols containing a four-ring carbon structure with a carbon side chain

d. a type of artery disease characterized by placques (accumulations of lipid-containing material) on the inner walls of the arteries

e. molecules of glycerol with one fatty acid attached

f. clusters of lipids associated with proteins that serve as transport vehicles for lipids in the lymph and blood

g. the class of lipoproteins that transport lipids from the intestinal cells to the rest of the body

h. the type of lipoprotein that transports cholesterol back to the liver from the cells; composed primarily of protein

i. the body's fat tissue; consists of masses of triglyceride-storing cells

j. fatty acids needed by the body but not made by it in amounts sufficient to meet physiological needs

Sample Test Questions

Select the best answer for each question.

1. Fats belong to a larger chemical classification known as:
   a. lipases.
   b. lecithins.
   c. labiles.
   d. leucines.
   e. lipids.

2. Of the lipids in foods and in the body, which are most abundant?
   a. Triglycerides
   b. Phospholipids
   c. Sterols
   b. Fatty acids

64

3. Fatty acids and triglycerides are composed of which atoms?
   a. Carbon, hydrogen, nitrogen
   b. Carbon, nitrogen, helium
   c. Hydrogen, mercury, oxygen
   d. Carbon, hydrogen, oxygen

4. Triglycerides are composed of:
   a. glycerol.
   b. choline.
   c. fatty acids.
   d. a and c
   e. b and c

5. The position of the double bond nearest the methyl group is described by a(n) _____ number.
   a. omega
   b. alpha
   c. delta
   d. polyunsaturated

6. Oleic acid has one double bond in the carbon chain. This means it is classified as:
   a. saturated.
   b. monounsaturated.
   c. diunsaturated.
   d. polyunsaturated.

7. The degree of unsaturation influences a fat's:
   a. stability.
   b. firmness.
   c. vulnerability to oxidation.
   d. all of the above

8. At room temperature, which type of fat is usually solid?
   a. Unsaturated fat
   b. Saturated fat
   c. Polyunsaturated fatty acid
   d. Omega-6 fatty acid

9. A disadvantage of hydrogenation is:
   a. the fats become resistant to oxidation.
   b. *cis*-fatty acids result.
   c. *trans*-fatty acids result.
   d. a and b
   e. b and c

10. Hydrogenation of fat renders it:
    a. more nutritious.
    b. more susceptible to oxidation and rancidity.
    c. less susceptible to oxidation and rancidity.
    d. less saturated, and thus less stable.

11. The manufacturing process that makes polyunsaturated fats more solid is called:
    a. centrifugation.
    b. hydrogenation.
    c. emulsification.
    d. modification.
    e. solidification.

12. The dispersion and stabilization of fat droplets in a watery solution is:
    a. hydrogenation.
    b. emulsification.
    c. saturation.
    d. precipitation.

13. Lecithin is a:
    a. carbohydrate.
    b. triglyceride.
    c. protein.
    d. phospholipid.

14. Which of the following is a compound with a multiple-ring structure?
    a. A phospholipid
    b. A sterol
    c. Glycerol
    d. A fatty acid

15. Cholesterol that is made in the body is:
    a. undesirable.
    b. only found in bile acids.
    c. exogenous.
    d. endogenous.

16. Bile is made from:
    a. glucose.
    b. cholesterol.
    c. vitamin D.
    d. prostaglandins.

17. A lipoprotein may be described as:
    a. a molecule made up of various amino acids.
    b. a triglyceride made of glycerol and three fatty acids.
    c. a cluster of lipids wrapped in a coat of protein.
    d. undigested fat circulating in the bloodstream.

18. The process of lipid absorption involves some molecules merging into spherical complexes called:
    a. micelles.
    b. bile.
    c. intestinal cells.
    d. lipoproteins.

19. The largest and least dense of the lipoproteins are the:
    a. chylomicrons.
    b. LDL.
    c. VLDL.
    d. HDL.

20. The lipoprotein thought to protect against coronary heart disease is:
    a. LDL.
    b. VLDL.
    c. IDL.
    d. HDL.
    e. the chylomicron.

21. The primary member of the omega-3 family is:
    a. lecithin.
    b. an eicosanoid.
    c. linolenic acid.
    d. linoleic acid.

22. Which of the following is a well-established and significant risk factor for cancer?
    a. Dietary fat
    b. Smoking
    c. Omega-3 fat intake
    d. Dietary cholesterol

23. Which enzyme hydrolyzes triglycerides from lipoproteins?
    a. Lipoprotein lipase (LPL)
    b. Hormone-sensitive lipase (HSL)
    c. Insulin lipase (IL)
    d. Lipoprotein protease (LPP)

24. Fat supplies what percentage of the body's ongoing energy needs during rest?
    a. 30%
    b. 40%
    c. 50%
    d. 60%

25. The lipid in food that influences blood cholesterol the most is:
    a. cholesterol.
    b. saturated fat.
    c. unsaturated fat.
    d. polyunsaturated fat.

26. Which of the following foods contains an appreciable amount of *trans* fat?
    a. Skim milk
    b. Bread
    c. Cakes and cookies
    d. Vegetables
    e. Fruits

27. Which contains the most saturated fat?
    a. Sunflower seed oil
    b. Corn oil
    c. Lard
    d. Olive oil

28. Which of the following foods contains no cholesterol?
    a. Beef steak
    b. Bacon
    c. Ice cream
    d. Baked potato

66

29. A change from whole milk to nonfat milk would:
    a. decrease the amount of fat and kcalories.
    b. increase the number of kcalories.
    c. increase satiety value of the meal.
    d. decrease the amount of protein.

30. Fat replacers that offer the desirable qualities of fat without the kcalories are:
    a. triglycerides.   c. artificial fats.
    b. chemical fats.   d. hydrogenated fats.

Short Answer Questions

1. The lipids include:

    a.   c.

    b.

2. Triglycerides are made of:

    a.   b.

3. Three ways that fatty acids differ from one another are:

    a.   c.

    b.

4. Three roles of phospholipids in the body are:

    a.

    b.

    c.

5. Four important sterols in the body are:

    a.   c.

    b.   d.

6. After bile enters the small intestine and emulsifies fat, what are its two possible destinations?

    a.

    b.

7. Four lipoproteins are:

    a.   c.

    b.   d.

8. Four roles of lipids in the body are:

    a.   c.

    b.   d.

9. Two essential fatty acids are:

    a.   b.

10. Three diseases associated with high saturated fat, *trans* fat, and cholesterol intakes are:

    a.   c.

    b.

11. Five major sources of monounsaturated fats are:

    a.   d.

    b.   e.

    c.

12. Three heart-healthy ways to prepare fish are:

    a.   c.

    b.

Problem Solving

1. Calculate the number of kcalories from fat for a person with a total energy intake of 2,000 kcalories who consumes 35% of kcalories from fat.

2. In the above problem, how many grams of fat would be consumed?

3. Your kcalorie needs are 2200 kcalories per day. How many kcalories should come from saturated fat?

4. In the above problem, how many grams of saturated fat would be consumed if you ate the maximum recommended?

5. Your kcalorie needs are 1700 kcalories per day and you are striving to consume a diet that provides 30% of your kcalories from fat. How many kcalories from fat must you consume?

6. In the above problem, how many grams of fat would you ingest?

7. You have prepared a milkshake that includes 2 cups of whole milk with ½ cup strawberries. How many grams of fat are in this product? How many kcalories from fat are in the milkshake?

8. In the above question, what percentage of the Daily Value for total fat will this milkshake provide?

68

9. You are considering eating a piece of pecan pie that provides 400 kcalories from fat. How many grams of fat does this dessert provide?

10. If your energy requirement is 1600 kcalories per day, what percentage of your fat allotment will the pie provide, assuming you are trying to eat 35% of total kcalories from fat each day?

Figure Identification

Identify these chemical structures.

1.

2.

3.

4.

5.

6.

❧ Chapter 5 Answer Key ❧

Summing Up

1. triglycerides
2. glycerol
3. unsaturation
4. location
5. saturated
6. double bonds
7. polyunsaturated
8. fatty acid
9. storage
10. saturated
11. oxidation
12. solid
13. *trans*
14. damage
15. soluble
16. emulsifiers
17. membranes
18. Sterols
19. cholesterol
20. absorb
21. bile
22. monoglycerides
23. chylomicrons
24. cells
25. lipids
26. lipoproteins
27. chylomicrons
28. triglycerides
29. half
30. cholesterol
31. protein
32. heart
33. protective
34. structural
35. essential
36. eicosanoids
37. immune
38. deficiencies
39. fat
40. nutrients
41. heart
42. low
43. monounsaturated
44. cancer
45. omega-3
46. food.

Chapter Study Questions

1. Triglycerides, phospholipids, sterols. Functions: triglycerides carry fat-soluble vitamins, induce satiety, provide the body with a continuous energy supply, keep the body warm, protect it from mechanical shock, and serve as starting materials for hormones; phospholipids and sterols contribute to cells' structures; cholesterol serves as raw material for hormones, vitamin D, and bile. Features: fats enhance foods' aroma and flavor, increase palatability, and provide kcalories and fat-soluble vitamins.

2. Essentiality and nonessentiality; size indicated by number of carbons; degree of saturation/unsaturation as indicated by the number of double bonds; location of double bonds in unsaturated fatty acids.

3. In polyunsaturated fatty acids, "omega" refers to the position of the first double bond relative to the methyl end of the chain. A polyunsaturated fatty acid with its closest double bond 3 carbons away from the methyl end is an omega-3 fatty acid. An omega-6 fatty acid is a polyunsaturated fatty acid with its closest double bond six carbons away from the methyl end.

4. Saturated fats have all their carbon atoms loaded with hydrogen atoms and contains only single bonds between its C atoms. Unsaturated fats have hydrogens removed, resulting in double bonds between carbon atoms; monounsaturated fats have two hydrogens removed and one double bond, whereas polyunsaturated fats have three or more double bonds and several hydrogens missing. Structurally, a triglyceride consists of a "backbone" of glycerol with three fatty acids attached.

5. Hydrogenation adds hydrogens to unsaturated fats to reduce the number of double bonds and make the fats more saturated and resistant to oxidation. Hydrogenation can increase a product's shelf life and add a desirable texture. Partial hydrogenation of unsaturated fats creates *trans*-fatty acids. A *trans*-fatty acid is one in which the hydrogens next to the double bonds are on opposite sides of the carbon chain. *Trans*-fatty acids are associated with increased heart disease risk and thus experts advise that intakes of these fatty acids be as limited as possible.

6. Phospholipids have a phosphate group (a phosphorus-containing salt) and choline (or another nitrogen-containing compound) in place of one of the fatty acids. This structure combines hydrophobic fatty acids (which dissolve in fat) with a hydrophilic phosphate group, enabling them to function as emulsifiers in the body. Cholesterol is a sterol, and its C, H, and O atoms are arranged in rings. Cholesterol in the body can serve as starting material for many important body compounds because of its structure.

7. Phospholipids are important parts of cell membranes, they help fat-soluble substances such as vitamins and hormones move back and forth across the cell membranes into the watery fluids on both sides, and they serve as emulsifiers to help suspend lipids in the blood and other body fluids. Cholesterol's vital roles are many, including serving as part of cell membranes, bile acids, sex hormones, adrenal hormones, and vitamin D.

8. A minimal amount of fat digestion occurs in the mouth and stomach via the actions of lingual lipase and gastric lipase, respectively. In the small intestine, bile emulsifies fats, allowing pancreatic and intestinal lipases to gain access to the fat for digestion, and the resulting fatty acids, monoglycerides, and other molecules are absorbed into intestinal cells. Within these cells, the products of lipid digestion are packaged with protein for transport. Cholesterol shuttles back and forth between the liver and the body cells in lipoproteins, and it also visits the intestinal tract in the form of bile.

9. Composed of triglycerides, cholesterol, phospholipids, and proteins, lipoproteins transport lipids in the body. Chylomicrons are the largest of the lipoproteins, formed in the intestinal wall following fat absorption, and they contain mostly triglycerides. VLDL are made in the liver and contain mostly triglycerides; LDL contain few triglycerides but are about half cholesterol. All three deliver lipids to body cells. HDL are about half protein and transport cholesterol back to the liver from body cells.

10. Linolenic acid (sources: plant oils, nuts, seeds, and vegetables such as soybeans) and linoleic acid (sources: seeds, nuts, vegetable oils, and poultry fat).

11. Excessive fat intake can contribute to weight gain and possibly promote growth of existing cancers. High saturated and *trans* fat intakes can contribute to elevated blood cholesterol and other blood lipids (and therefore heart disease). Some saturated fats raise total cholesterol and LDL; *trans*-fatty acids raise LDL and lower HDL. Soluble dietary fibers, phytochemicals, moderate alcohol consumption, and physical activity may lower LDL and/or raise HDL.

12. Consume a diet that is low in saturated fat (<10% of energy intake), *trans* fat (as little as possible), and cholesterol (≤300 mg/day). Limit total fat intake to 20% to 35% of daily energy.

13. Replacing saturated fat with unsaturated fat reduces LDL cholesterol and lowers risk of heart disease. Regular intake of omega-3 polyunsaturated fatty acids helps prevent blood clots, protect against irregular heartbeats, improve blood lipids, lower blood pressure, support healthy immune function, and suppress inflammation. Omega-3 fats from fish may protect against some cancers.

14. The Daily Values (which are used to calculate the %DV on food labels) are 65 grams total fat and 20 grams saturated fat. For a person who consumes 2000 kcalories a day, these numbers represent intakes roughly equivalent to 30% of kcal from fat and 10% of kcal from saturated fat.

15. Consume 20-35% of total energy from primarily mono- and polyunsaturated fats; limit saturated fat intake to 10% or less of kcal, and minimize *trans* fat intake. Restrict cholesterol intake to 300 mg or less per day. In practice, this means consuming a mostly plant-based diet emphasizing unsaturated fat sources such as non-tropical plant oils, nuts, seeds, and fatty fish; and limiting solid fats, processed or fast foods made with hydrogenated fats, fatty meats, and whole-milk products.

Key Terms Practice

1. fats	8. choline	16. d	24. b
2. plaque	9. sterols	17. g	25. j
3. A: lipases;	10. b	18. j	26. h
D: lecithin	11. f	19. e	27. f
4. glycerol	12. i	20. i	28. e
5. micelles	13. c	21. d	29. a
6. lipids	14. h	22. c	
7. oils	15. a	23. g	

Sample Test Questions

1. e (p. 129)	9. c (p. 135)	17. c (p. 141)	25. b (p. 147)
2. a (p. 129)	10. c (pp. 134-135)	18. a (p. 140)	26. c (p. 148)
3. d (p. 129)	11. b (p. 134)	19. a (p. 141)	27. c (p. 148)
4. d (p. 130)	12. b (p. 136)	20. d (p. 143)	28. d (p. 137)
5. a (p. 132)	13. d (p. 136)	21. c (p. 145)	29. a (p. 153)
6. b (p. 131)	14. b (p. 137)	22. b (p. 148)	30. c (p. 155)
7. d (pp. 133-134)	15. d (p. 137)	23. a (p. 146)	
8. b (p. 133)	16. b (p. 137)	24. d (p. 146)	

Short Answer Questions

1. triglycerides, phospholipids, sterols
2. glycerol, 3 fatty acids
3. carbon chain length, number of double bonds, location of double bonds
4. serving as constituents of cell membranes; helping fat-soluble substances pass easily in and out of cells; acting as emulsifiers in the body
5. cholesterol, bile acids, vitamin D, sex and adrenal hormones
6. reabsorbed from the small intestine and recycled; trapped by dietary fibers in large intestine and excreted
7. chylomicrons, VLDL, LDL, HDL
8. provide energy; insulate against temperature extremes; protect against shock; maintain cell membranes
9. linoleic acid, linolenic acid
10. heart disease, cancer, obesity
11. olive oil, canola oil, peanut oil, safflower oil, avocados
12. grilling, baking, broiling

Problem Solving

1. 2,000 kcal × 0.35 = 700 kcalories

2. 700 kcal divided by 9 kcal/g = 78 grams

3. 2200 kcal × 0.10 = 220 kcalories or less (saturated fats are not essential nutrients)

4. 220 kcal divided by 9 kcal/g = 24 grams

5. 1700 kcal × 0.30 = 510 kcalories from fat

6. 510 kcal divided by 9 kcal/g = 57 grams of fat

7. 2 cups milk × 8 grams fat/cup = 16 grams of fat
   16 g × 9 kcal/g = 144 kcalories from fat

8. 16 grams divided by 65 grams fat = 25% of Daily Value for fat

9. 400 kcal divided by 9 kcal/g = 44 grams of fat

10. 1600 kcal × 0.35 = 560 kcalories per day from fat
    560 kcal divided by 9 kcal/g = 62 total grams of fat
    44 g divided by 62 g = 71% from the pie   *or* 400 kcal divided by 560 kcal = 71%

Figure Identification

1. glycerol
2. a saturated fatty acid (stearic acid)
3. a polyunsaturated fatty acid (linoleic acid)
4. linoleic acid (an omega-6 fatty acid)
5. linolenic acid (an omega-3 fatty acid)
6. cholesterol

⑥ Chapter 6 ~ Protein: Amino Acids ⑥

Chapter Outline

I. The Chemist's View of Proteins
  A. Amino Acids
    1. Unique Side Groups
    2. Nonessential Amino Acids
    3. Essential Amino Acids
    4. Conditionally Essential Amino Acids
  B. Proteins
    1. Amino Acid Chains
    2. Primary Structure—Amino Acid Sequence
    3. Secondary Structure—Polypeptide Shapes
    4. Tertiary Structure—Polypeptide Tangles
    5. Quaternary Structures—Multiple Polypeptide Interactions
    6. Protein Denaturation
II. Digestion and Absorption of Proteins
  A. Protein Digestion
    1. In the Stomach
    2. In the Small Intestine
  B. Protein Absorption
III. Proteins in the Body
  A. Protein Synthesis
    1. Delivering the Instructions
    2. Lining Up the Amino Acids
    3. Sequencing Errors
    4. Gene Expression
  B. Roles of Proteins
    1. As Structural Materials
    2. As Enzymes
    3. As Hormones
    4. As Regulators of Fluid Balance
    5. As Acid-Base Regulators
    6. As Transporters
    7. As Antibodies
    8. As a Source of Energy and Glucose
    9. Other Roles
  C. A Preview of Protein Metabolism
    1. Protein Turnover and the Amino Acid Pool
    2. Nitrogen Balance

    3. Using Amino Acids to Make Other Compounds
    4. Using Amino Acids for Energy and Glucose
    5. Using Amino Acids to Make Fat
    6. Deaminating Amino Acids
    7. Using Amino Acids to Make Proteins and Nonessential Amino Acids
    8. Converting Ammonia to Urea
    9. Excreting Urea
IV. Protein in Foods
  A. Protein Quality
    1. Digestibility
    2. Amino Acid Composition
    3. Reference Protein
    4. High-Quality Proteins
  B. Complementary Proteins
V. Health Effects and Recommended Intakes of Protein
  A. Health Effects of Protein
    1. Protein Deficiency
    2. Heart Disease
    3. Cancer
    4. Adult Bone Loss (Osteoporosis)
    5. Weight Control
    6. Kidney Disease
  B. Recommended Intakes of Protein
    1. Protein RDA
    2. Adequate Energy
  C. From Guidelines to Groceries
    1. Protein Foods
    2. Milk and Milk Products
    3. Fruits, Vegetables, and Grains
  D. Read Food Labels
  E. Protein and Amino Acid Supplements
    1. Protein Powders
    2. Amino Acid Supplements
VI. Nutritional Genomics
  A. A Genomics Primer
  B. Genetic Variation and Disease
    1. Single-Gene Disorders
    2. Multigene Disorders
  C. Clinical Concerns

Summing Up

Chemically speaking, proteins are more 1._____ than carbohydrates or lipids; they are made of some 20 different amino acids, 9 of which the body cannot make (the 2._____ amino acids). Each amino acid contains an 3._____ _____, an acid group, a hydrogen atom, and a distinctive 4._____ group,

all attached to a central carbon atom. Peptide bonds link amino acids together in a series of
5._____ reactions to create proteins. The distinctive sequence of amino acids in each protein
determines its unique shape and 6._____.

Digestion is facilitated mostly by the stomach's acid and 7._____, which first denature dietary
proteins, then cleave them into smaller 8._____ and some amino acids. Pancreatic and
intestinal enzymes split these polypeptides further, to oligo-, tri-, and 9._____, and then split most
of these to single amino acids. Then carriers in the membranes of intestinal cells 10._____ the
amino acids into the cells, where they are released into the bloodstream.

Cells synthesize proteins according to genetic information that dictates the 11._____ in which
amino acids are linked together. Each protein plays a specific role. Body proteins function as structural materials, as
12._____, as hormones, in 13._____ and acid-base balance, as transporters, as
14._____, and to provide energy and glucose, among other roles.

Proteins are constantly being 15._____ and broken down as needed. The body's
assimilation of amino acids into proteins and its release of amino acids via protein breakdown and
16._____ can be tracked by measuring 17._____ balance, which should be positive
during growth and steady in adulthood. An energy deficit or an inadequate protein intake may force the body to use
amino acids as 18._____, creating a 19._____ nitrogen balance. Protein eaten in excess of need is
degraded and stored as body 20._____.

A diet that supplies all of the essential amino acids in adequate amounts ensures protein
21._____. The best guarantee of amino acid adequacy is to eat foods containing 22._____-
_____ proteins or mixtures of foods containing 23._____ proteins that can each
supply the amino acids missing in the other. In addition to its amino acid content, the quality of protein is measured
by its 24._____ and its ability to support 25._____. Such measures are of great
importance in dealing with 26._____ worldwide, but in countries where protein deficiency is
not common, the protein quality of individual foods deserves little 27._____.

Protein deficiency impairs the body's ability to grow and 28._____ optimally. Excesses of protein
offer no advantage; in fact, overconsumption of protein-rich foods may incur health 29._____ as well.
The optimal diet is adequate in energy from carbohydrate and fat and delivers 30._____ grams of protein per
kilogram of healthy body weight each day. U.S. and Canadian diets are typically 31._____ than adequate in this
respect. Normal, healthy people do not need protein or amino acid 32._____.

Chapter Study Questions

1. How does the chemical structure of proteins differ from the structures of carbohydrates and fats?

74

2. Describe the structure of amino acids, and explain how their sequence in proteins affects the proteins' shapes. What are the essential amino acids?

3. Describe protein digestion and absorption.

4. Can taking enzyme supplements improve a person's digestion? Explain why or why not.

5. Describe protein synthesis.

6. Describe some of the roles proteins play in the human body.

7. What are enzymes? What roles do they play in chemical reactions? What are hormones?

8. How does the body use amino acids? What is deamination? Define nitrogen balance. What conditions are associated with zero, positive, and negative balance?

9. What factors affect the quality of dietary protein? What is a high-quality protein?

10. How can vegetarians meet their protein needs without eating meat?

11. What are the health consequences of ingesting inadequate protein and energy?

12. How might protein excess influence health?

13. What factors are considered in establishing recommended protein intakes?

14. What are the benefits and risks of taking protein and amino acid supplements?

Key Terms Practice

To complete the crossword puzzle, identify the key term that best matches each definition.

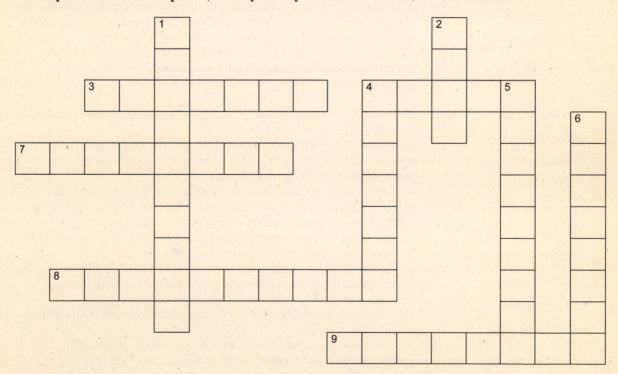

Across:
3. A compound with the chemical formula NH_3; produced during the deamination of amino acids.
4. The swelling of body tissue caused by excessive amounts of fluid in the interstitial spaces; seen in protein deficiency (among other conditions).

76

7. Substances that elicit the formation of antibodies or an inflammation reaction from the immune system.
8. Large proteins of the blood and body fluids, produced by the immune system in response to the invasion of the body by foreign molecules.
9. Higher-than-normal acidity in the blood and body fluids.

Down:
1. The globular protein of the red blood cells that carries oxygen from the lungs to the cells throughout the body.
2. The principal nitrogen-excretion product of protein metabolism.
4. Proteins that facilitate chemical reactions without being changed in the process; protein catalysts.
5. Higher-than-normal alkalinity (base) in the blood and body fluids.
6. Compounds composed of carbon, hydrogen, oxygen, and nitrogen atoms, arranged into amino acids linked in a chain.

Match the key terms with their definitions.

10. _____ amino acids

11. _____ conditionally essential amino acid

12. _____ denaturation

13. _____ essential amino acids

14. _____ limiting amino acid

15. _____ nonessential amino acids

16. _____ peptidase

17. _____ peptide bond

18. _____ polypeptide

19. _____ transcription

a. building blocks of proteins containing an amino group, an acid group, a hydrogen atom, and a distinctive side group, all attached to a central carbon atom
b. amino acids that the body can synthesize
c. amino acids that the body cannot synthesize in amounts sufficient to meet physiological needs
d. an amino acid that is normally not essential, but must be supplied by the diet in special circumstances when the need for it exceeds the body's ability to produce it
e. a bond that connects the acid end of one amino acid with the amino end of another, forming a link in a protein chain
f. many (ten or more) amino acids bonded together
g. the change in a protein's shape and consequent loss of its function brought about by heat, agitation, acid, base, alcohol, heavy metals, or other agents
h. a digestive enzyme that hydrolyzes peptide bonds
i. the process of messenger RNA being made from a template of DNA
j. the essential amino acid found in the shortest supply relative to the amounts needed for protein synthesis in the body

20. _____ amino acid pool

21. _____ deamination

22. _____ gene expression

23. _____ high-quality proteins

24. _____ neurotransmitters

25. _____ nitrogen balance

26. _____ protein digestibility

27. _____ protein turnover

28. _____ transamination

29. _____ translation

a. the process of messenger RNA directing the sequence of amino acids and synthesis of proteins
b. the process by which a cell converts the genetic code into RNA and protein
c. the degradation and synthesis of protein
d. the supply of amino acids derived from either food proteins or body proteins that collect in the cells and circulating blood and stand ready to be incorporated in proteins and other compounds or used for energy
e. the amount of nitrogen consumed (N in) as compared with the amount of nitrogen excreted (N out) in a given period of time
f. chemicals that are released at the end of a nerve cell when a nerve impulse arrives there; they diffuse across the gap to the next cell and alter the membrane of that second cell to either inhibit or excite it
g. removal of the amino (NH_2) group from a compound such as an amino acid
h. the transfer of an amino group from one amino acid to a keto acid, producing a new nonessential amino acid and a new keto acid
i. dietary proteins containing all the essential amino acids in relatively the same amounts that human beings require
j. a measure of the amount of amino acids absorbed from a given protein intake

Sample Test Questions

Select the best answer for each question.

1. Proteins differ from the other energy nutrients in that they contain:
   a. glycerol.
   b. carbon.
   c. oxygen.
   d. nitrogen.

2. A polypeptide is:
   a. many amino acids linked together by peptide bonds.
   b. formation of a helix by adenine, thymine, guanine, and cystosine.
   c. the secondary structure of an amino acid.
   d. composed of glucose and amino acids.

3. The structures of amino acids differ in that:
   a. some do not contain nitrogen.
   b. some do not contain carbon.
   c. they each have a different side group.
   d. they each have different acid groups.

4. When an enzyme is used in a chemical reaction in the body, it:
   a. forms ATP.
   b. remains unchanged.
   c. is degraded into a substance containing less chemical energy.
   d. only breaks down substances.

5. Proteins maintain acid-base balance in the body by:
   a. acting as buffers.
   b. secreting chloride ions.
   c. secreting acids.
   d. tying up excess sodium ions.

6.-11. Match the following:

6. _____ enzyme
7. _____ antibody
8. _____ hormone
9. _____ opsin
10. _____ antigen
11. _____ fluid balance

   a. elicits the formation of antibodies
   b. protein catalyst
   c. inactivates foreign agents
   d. a chemical messenger
   e. maintenance of proper fluids in body compartments
   f. visual pigment protein

12. Methionine, threonine, and tryptophan are names of:
   a. proteins.
   b. fatty acids.
   c. essential amino acids.
   d. lipids.
   e. nonessential amino acids.

13. If an essential amino acid required for formation of a certain enzyme is missing in the diet:
   a. another amino acid will be substituted in its place so the enzyme can be made.
   b. synthesis of the enzyme will stop.
   c. the partially synthesized enzyme will be stored in the adipose tissue until the missing amino acid is supplied in the diet.
   d. the amino acid will be made from glucose.

14. In the stomach, protein digestion is facilitated by:
   a. hydrochloric acid.
   b. pepsin.
   c. pancreatic enzymes.
   d. a and b

15. The process of messenger RNA being made from a template of DNA is:
   a. transcription.
   b. translation.
   c. amino acid oxidation.
   d. messenger RNA replication.

16. Instructions for making proteins are found within the cell's:
    a. protein strand.
    b. ribosomes.
    c. RNA.
    d. DNA.

17. The making of specific types of proteins in certain amounts and at certain rates is called:
    a. epigenetics.
    b. replication.
    c. gene expression.
    d. translation.

18. An excess of interstitial fluid can cause:
    a. intravascular storage.
    b. edema.
    c. alkalosis.
    d. protein reabsorption.

19. The body can normally detect invading disease-causing substances, which are called:
    a. antibodies.
    b. buffers.
    c. a matrix.
    d. antigens.

20. If the body degrades more protein than it synthesizes and loses protein, nitrogen balance becomes:
    a. nitrogen output.
    b. negative.
    c. zero.
    d. positive.

21. When amino acids are used for energy, they are broken down. This is called:
    a. deamination.
    b. amination.
    c. neurotransmitter formation.
    d. positive nitrogen balance.

22. The quality of a food protein:
    a. is evaluated using the amino acid requirements of preschool-aged children.
    b. is partially determined by its amino acid composition.
    c. is based on comparison with a reference protein.
    d. a and b
    e. b and c
    f. a, b, and c

23. Which foods contain high-quality proteins?
    a. Eggs, meat, fish, corn, and seeds
    b. Eggs, meat, poultry, soy, and milk
    c. Eggs, meat, fish, gelatin, and grains
    d. Meat, milk, cheese, corn, and spinach

24. Protein eaten in excess is stored as:
    a. muscle.
    b. bone.
    c. glycogen.
    d. fat.
    e. all of the above

25. Protein deficiency causes:
    a. slowed growth.
    b. impaired brain and kidney functions.
    c. poor immunity.
    d. all of the above

26. Excessive animal protein intake can be a factor in the following conditions:
    a. heart disease, cancer, and osteoporosis.
    b. heart disease, anorexia, and cancer.
    c. heart disease, kidney disease, and liver disease.
    d. cancer, osteoporosis, and dental caries.

27. The protein RDA for adults is:
    a. 0.8 g per pound of body weight.
    b. 0.8 g per kg of body weight.
    c. 1.2 g per pound body weight.
    d. 1.5 g per kg body weight.

28. When establishing the protein RDA, the committee assumed:
    a. that people have unusual metabolic needs for protein.
    b. that the protein consumed will be of high quality.
    c. that protein will be consumed along with sufficient carbohydrate and fat.
    d. all of the above

29. Amino acid supplements:
    a. can cure herpes.
    b. can facilitate weight loss.
    c. can strengthen fingernails.
    d. can be harmful.

30. Large doses of branched-chain amino acids may:
    a. lower plasma concentrations of ammonia.
    b. improve athletic performance.
    c. raise ammonia levels, which may be toxic to the brain.
    d. provide more fuel than fatty acids.

Short Answer Questions

1. The atoms found in all proteins are:

    a.   c.

    b.   d.

2. The three common parts of all amino acids are:

    a.   c.

    b.   d.

3. Two compounds in the stomach that help to digest proteins are:

    a.   b.

4. Functions of proteins (other than providing energy) include:

    a.   f.

    b.   g.

    c.   h.

    d.   i.

    e.   j.

5. Two products that result from deamination are:

    a.   b.

6. The quality of dietary protein depends on its:

    a.   b.

7. Combining complementary amino acids at each meal is not necessary for vegetarians if they:

    a.

    b.

8. Problems associated with intake of excess protein from red and processed meats include:

    a.   b.

80

9. Potential adverse effects of amino acid supplements include:

   a.

   b.

   c.

Problem Solving

1. Based on the DRI recommendations, how many kcalories should come from protein in a 1700-kcal diet (provide range)?

2. How many grams of protein should contribute to the above recommendation?

3. If a meal provides a total of 570 kcalories, and 130 of those kcalories are from protein, what percentage of the kcalories come from protein?

4. What is the protein requirement for a person whose appropriate weight is 176 lb.?

5. A person's total kcalorie requirement is 2500. If this person consumes 950 kcalories from protein, what percent of kcalories are from protein?

6. How many grams of protein did the person in the previous question consume?

7. Is this amount within the recommended range for protein intake?

8. If a person's protein requirement is 175 grams per day, how many kcalories should be consumed from protein?

9. If a person's protein requirement is 75 grams per day, what is the person's body weight in kg and in pounds?

10. If a person weighs 165 pounds, how many grams of protein should the person consume daily?

Figure Identification

Identify these structures and reaction.

1.

2.

3.

4.

꩜ **Chapter 6 Answer Key** ꩜

Summing Up

1. complex
2. essential
3. amino group
4. side
5. condensation
6. function
7. enzymes
8. polypeptides
9. dipeptides
10. transport
11. sequence
12. enzymes
13. fluid
14. antibodies
15. synthesized
16. excretion
17. nitrogen
18. fuel
19. negative
20. fat
21. synthesis
22. high-quality
23. complementary
24. digestibility
25. growth
26. malnutrition
27. emphasis
28. function
29. problems
30. 0.8
31. more
32. supplements

Chapter Study Questions

1. Like carbohydrates and fats, proteins contain carbon, hydrogen, and oxygen, but proteins also contain nitrogen. Proteins are composed of chains of compounds called amino acids, often folded once or many times into unique shapes. Each of the ~20 amino acids that appear in body proteins is different from the others thanks to its distinct side chain, making protein structures much more complex and varied than those of carbohydrates or fats.

2. An amino acid molecule consists of a central carbon atom with an amino group (NH_2), a hydrogen atom, an acid group (COOH), and a unique side group (which can be a single atom or a compound) bonded to it. Amino acids are linked together by peptide bonds to form polypeptides, the primary structure of proteins. Amino acid side chains are attracted to or repelled from various other amino acids and the water in body fluids, so the polypeptide chain is twisted around as a result of these attractive/repulsive forces. For instance, the protein shape may be arranged to keep hydrophilic side groups to the exterior of the protein, and hydrophobic side groups facing inward. The sequence and special characteristics of the side chains thus help determine the protein's shape. The essential amino acids are those the body cannot synthesize in amounts sufficient to meet physiological needs, including: histidine, isoleucine, leucine, lysine, methionine, phenylalanine, threonine, tryptophan, and valine.

3. In the mouth, chewing and crushing moisten protein-rich foods and mix them with saliva to be swallowed. In the stomach, stomach acid uncoils protein strands and activates enzymes; pepsin and HCl break protein down into smaller polypeptides. In the small intestine, pancreatic and small intestinal enzymes split polypeptides further into dipeptides, tripeptides, and amino acids, and then enzymes on the surface of the small intestinal cells hydrolyze most of the peptides. The intestinal cells absorb the amino acids and some di- and tripeptides using a number of specific carriers.

4. Enzymes in supplements offer no digestive assistance or benefit because they are digested to amino acids, just as all proteins are. Even the digestive enzymes—which function optimally at their specific pH—are denatured and digested when the pH of their environment changes.

5. DNA in the nucleus of each cell serves as a template to make strands of messenger RNA. Each messenger RNA strand carries instructions for some protein the cell needs; the messenger RNA leaves the nucleus, and attaches itself to the protein-making machinery of the cell (ribosome). Transfer RNA carry amino acids to the messenger RNA, which dictates the sequence in which they will snap into place; this lines up the amino acids in sequence. The amino acids are then linked together in sequence by enzymes, the completed protein strand is released, and the transfer RNA are re-used.

6. Proteins form the structural materials of body cells and tissues (muscles, blood, skin, bone, etc.), serve as enzymes (catalysts), regulate body processes as hormones, help maintain the body's fluid balance by attracting water, help maintain acid-base balance by acting as buffers, transport nutrients and other molecules into and out of cells and within body fluids, act against disease agents as antibodies, provide a source of energy and glucose (especially when dietary carbohydrate is inadequate), help clot blood, help make scar tissue, and serve as light-sensitive visual pigments.

7. Enzymes are protein catalysts that facilitate the synthesis of larger compounds from smaller ones and hydrolysis of larger compounds to smaller ones without being affected in the process. Hormones are chemical messengers that are secreted by a variety of endocrine glands in response to altered conditions in the body.

8. The body uses amino acids to synthesize proteins, nonessential amino acids, and other compounds such as neurotransmitters (norepinephrine and epinephrine), melanin, and hormones such as thyroxin. Amino acids may also be used to produce energy, glucose, or fat. Deamination is removal of the amino group from a compound such as an amino acid. Nitrogen balance: the amount of nitrogen consumed compared with the amount of nitrogen excreted. Zero N balance: normal, healthy adults; positive N balance: growing children, pregnant women, and people recovering from protein deficiency or illness; negative N balance: people who are starving or in severe stress (e.g., because of burns, injuries, infections, or fever).

9. Its supply of a balance of the essential amino acids and its digestibility. A high-quality protein is a protein containing all the amino acids essential in human nutrition in relatively the same amounts required.

10. Vegetarians who eat animal products such as eggs and/or milk products obtain high-quality proteins from those foods. Strict vegetarians can obtain protein from legumes, nuts, vegetables, and whole grains. Strict vegetarians can combine plant protein foods that have different but complementary amino acid patterns.

11. Decreased protein synthesis and increased protein degradation, potentially leading to protein-energy malnutrition if severe. Protein deficiency causes poor growth in children, impaired brain and kidney functions, poor immunity, and inadequate nutrient absorption.

12. Diets too high in protein offer no benefits. They often contribute saturated fat-rich foods of animal origin that may contribute to the progression of heart disease. High-protein diets may promote calcium losses and deplete the bones of this mineral (especially if combined with low calcium intakes); if much animal-derived protein (e.g., red or processed meat) is eaten, this may contribute to the development of cancer. High-protein diets that are low in kcalories promote weight loss (just as all low-kcal diets do), but may be inadequate if healthful fruits, vegetables, and whole grains are restricted. Excess protein, though not harmful to the kidneys of healthy people, can stress these organs in those with chronic kidney disease, accelerating the decline in kidney function in these individuals.

13. The DRI Committee considers the need for protein to replace worn-out tissue or build new tissue during growth, and the typical quality of the protein eaten. The RDA is based on a diet adequate in kcalories and other nutrients and providing protein from mixed-quality sources. Many fitness authorities publish recommendations specifically for athletes that also consider the type of training regularly performed as well.

14. Whey protein supplements may increase protein synthesis slightly when consumed in conjunction with athletic training, but do not seem to improve performance; whey protein (and protein in general) is best consumed in foods. There are no proven benefits for amino acid supplements in healthy people, but risks include diarrhea, amino acid imbalances, and toxicities. Branched-chain amino acid supplements may benefit individuals with liver disease, but can raise plasma ammonia concentrations to potentially toxic levels when taken in large doses. Lysine may or may not suppress herpes infections, but its use appears to be safe at levels of up to 3 g/day if doses are divided among meals. Tryptophan may be effective for pain and insomnia relief, but taking tryptophan supplements may cause eosinophilia-myalgia syndrome (EMS). The amino acid arginine is thought to be protective against heart disease, and research to confirm this is underway; however, consumers are currently not recommended to take arginine supplements (unless they are prescribed by a physician).

Key Terms Practice

1. hemoglobin	8. antibodies	16. h	24. f
2. urea	9. acidosis	17. e	25. e
3. ammonia	10. a	18. f	26. j
4. A: edema;	11. d	19. i	27. c
D: enzymes	12. g	20. d	28. h
5. alkalosis	13. c	21. g	29. a
6. proteins	14. j	22. b	
7. antigens	15. b	23. i	

Sample Test Questions

1. d (p. 168)	9. f (p. 178)	17. c (p. 175)	25. d (p. 182)
2. a (p. 169)	10. a (p. 177)	18. b (p. 176)	26. a (pp. 182-183)
3. c (p. 168)	11. e (p. 176)	19. d (p. 177)	27. b (p. 184)
4. b (pp. 175-176)	12. c (pp. 168, 181)	20. b (p. 178)	28. c (p. 184)
5. a (p. 176)	13. b (p. 181)	21. a (p. 179)	29. d (p. 186-187)
6. b (p. 175)	14. d (pp. 171, 172)	22. f (p. 181)	30. c (p. 187)
7. c (p. 177)	15. a (p. 173)	23. b (p. 181)	
8. d (p. 176)	16. d (p. 173)	24. d (p. 179)	

Short Answer Questions

1. carbon, hydrogen, oxygen, nitrogen
2. central carbon (C), amino group (NH_2), acid group (COOH), hydrogen (H)
3. hydrochloric acid, pepsin
4. structural materials, enzymes, hormones, fluid balance, acid-base balance, transport proteins, antibodies, blood clotting, scar tissue formation, visual pigments
5. ammonia, keto acid
6. digestibility, amino acid composition
7. consume a varied protein intake; consume sufficient kcalories
8. heart disease, cancer
9. diarrhea; deficiencies or toxicities of specific amino acids; increased plasma ammonia concentrations

Problem Solving

1. $1700 \times 0.10 = 170$ kcalories
    $1700 \times 0.35 = 595$ kcalories
    170-595 kcalories

2. 170 kcal divided by 4 kcal/g = 43 grams
    595 kcal divided by 4 kcal/g = 149 grams
    43-149 grams of protein

3. 130 kcal divided by 570 kcal = 23%

4. 176 lb. divided by 2.2 lb./kg = 80 kg
    0.8 g/kg $\times$ 80 kg = 64 g protein per day

5. 950 divided by 2500 = 38%

6. 950 kcal divided by 4 kcal/g = 238 grams protein

7. Based on the AMDR of 10-35% of total energy intake, this amount (representing 38% of kcal) exceeds the recommendation for protein intake.

8. 175 g $\times$ 4 kcal/g = 700 kcalories

9. 75 g divided by 0.8 g/kg = 93.75 kg $\times$ 2.2 lb./kg = 206 pounds

10. 165 lb. divided by 2.2 lb./kg = 75 kg $\times$ 0.8 g/kg = 60 grams of protein

Figure Identification

1. amino acid structure
2. condensation of 2 amino acids to form a dipeptide
3. glycine
4. aspartic acid

❧ Chapter 7 ~ Energy Metabolism ❧

Chapter Outline

I. Chemical Reactions in the Body
  A. The Site of Metabolic Reactions—Cells
  B. The Building Reactions—Anabolism
  C. The Breakdown Reactions—Catabolism
  D. The Transfer of Energy in Reactions—ATP
  E. The Helpers in Metabolic Reactions—Enzymes and Coenzymes

II. Breaking Down Nutrients for Energy
  A. Glucose
    1. Glucose-to-Pyruvate
    2. Pyruvate's Options—Anaerobic or Aerobic
    3. Pyruvate-to-Lactate (Anaerobic)
    4. Pyruvate-to-Acetyl CoA (Aerobic)
  B. Glycerol and Fatty Acids
    1. Glycerol-to-Pyruvate
    2. Fatty Acids-to-Acetyl CoA
    3. Fatty Acids Cannot Make Glucose
  C. Amino Acids
    1. Amino Acid Deamination
    2. Amino Acid Pathways
  D. The Final Steps of Energy Metabolism
    1. The TCA Cycle
    2. The Electron Transport Chain

    3. The kCalories-per-Gram Secret Revealed
III. Feasting and Fasting
  A. Feasting—Excess Energy
    1. Excess Protein
    2. Excess Carbohydrate
    3. Excess Fat
  B. The Transition from Feasting to Fasting
  C. Fasting—Inadequate Energy
    1. Adaptation: Making Glucose
    2. Adaptation: Creating an Alternate Fuel
    3. Adaptation: Conserving Energy
  D. Low-Carbohydrate Diets
IV. Alcohol in the Body
  A. Alcohol in Beverages
  B. Alcohol's Influence
    1. In the GI Tract
    2. In the Liver
    3. In the Brain
  C. Alcohol's Damage
    1. Dehydration
    2. Malnutrition
    3. Short-Term Effects
    4. Long-Term Effects
  D. Personal Strategies

Summing Up

During digestion the energy-yielding nutrients—carbohydrates, fats, and proteins—are broken down to 1._____ (and other monosaccharides), glycerol, fatty acids, and 2._____ acids. With the help of enzymes and 3._____, the cells use these molecules to build more complex compounds (4._____) or break them down further to release energy (5._____). High-energy compounds such as 6._____ may capture the energy released during catabolism and provide the energy needed for 7._____.

The glucose-to-energy pathway begins with 8._____—the breakdown of glucose to 9._____. Pyruvate may be converted to 10._____ anaerobically or to 11._____ _____ aerobically. The pathway from pyruvate to acetyl CoA is 12._____. Once the commitment to acetyl CoA is made, 13._____ is not retrievable; acetyl CoA cannot go back to glucose. Glucose can be synthesized only from 14._____ or compounds earlier in the pathway.

The body can convert the small 15._____ portion of a triglyceride to either pyruvate (and then glucose) or acetyl CoA. The 16._____ _____ of a triglyceride, on the other hand, cannot make glucose, but they can provide abundant acetyl CoA. Acetyl CoA may then enter the 17._____ cycle to release energy or combine with other molecules of acetyl CoA to make body 18._____.

The body can use some amino acids to make 19._____, whereas others can be used either to provide energy or to make 20._____. Before an amino acid enters any of these metabolic pathways, its 21._____-containing amino group must be removed through 22._____.

Carbohydrate, fat, and protein take different paths to 23._____ _____, but once there, the final pathways—the TCA cycle and 24._____ transport chain—are shared. A living cell is busy during the metabolism of 25._____ of compounds, each of which may be involved in several reactions, each requiring an 26._____.

When energy intake 27._____ energy needs, the body makes fat—regardless of whether the excess intake is from 28._____, carbohydrate, or fat. The only difference is that the body is much more 29._____ at storing energy when the excess derives from dietary fat.

When fasting, the body makes a number of 30._____: increasing the breakdown of fat to provide 31._____ for most of the cells, using 32._____ and amino acids to make glucose for the red blood cells and central nervous system, producing 33._____ to fuel the brain, suppressing the appetite, and slowing 34._____. All of these measures conserve 35._____ and minimize losses. Low-carbohydrate diets incur similar changes in 36._____.

Chapter Study Questions

1. Define metabolism, anabolism, and catabolism; give an example of each.

2. Name one of the body's high-energy molecules, and describe how is it used.

3. What are coenzymes, and what service do they provide in metabolism?

4. Name the four basic units derived from foods that are used by the body in metabolic transformations. How many carbons are in the "backbones" of each?

5. Define aerobic and anaerobic metabolism. How does insufficient oxygen influence metabolism?

6. How does the body dispose of excess nitrogen?

7. Summarize the main steps in the metabolism of glucose, glycerol, fatty acids, and amino acids.

8. Describe how a surplus of the three energy nutrients contributes to body fat stores.

9. What adaptations does the body make during a fast? What are ketone bodies? Define ketosis.

10. Distinguish between a loss of fat and a loss of weight, and describe how both might happen.

Key Terms Practice

To complete the crossword puzzle, identify the key term that best matches each definition.

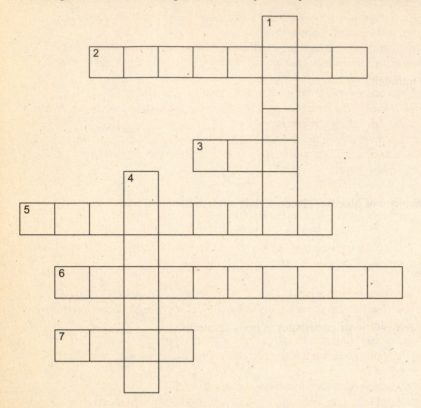

Across:
2. A 3-carbon compound that plays a key role in energy metabolism.
3. The coenzyme derived from the B vitamin pantothenic acid and central to energy metabolism.
5. Complex organic molecules that work with enzymes to facilitate the enzymes' activity.
6. The metabolic breakdown of glucose to pyruvate, which does not require oxygen.
7. Compounds that cells can use for energy.

Down:
1. A 3-carbon compound produced from pyruvate during anaerobic metabolism.
4. Proteins that act as catalysts, facilitating chemical reactions without being changed in the process.

Match the key terms with their definitions.

8. _____ acetyl CoA

9. _____ aerobic

10. _____ anaerobic

11. _____ adenosine triphosphate

12. _____ Cori cycle

13. _____ coupled reactions

14. _____ electron transport chain

15. _____ mitochondria

16. _____ photosynthesis

17. _____ tricarboxylic acid cycle

a. the process by which green plants use the sun's energy to make carbohydrates from carbon dioxide and water

b. a common high-energy compound composed of a purine (adenine), a sugar (ribose), and three phosphate groups

c. pairs of chemical reactions in which some of the energy released from the breakdown of one compound is used to create a bond in the formation of another compound

d. a 2-carbon compound to which a molecule of CoA is attached

e. a series of metabolic reactions that break down molecules of acetyl CoA to carbon dioxide and hydrogen atoms

f. the final pathway in energy metabolism that transports electrons from hydrogen to oxygen and captures the energy released in the bonds of ATP

g. not requiring oxygen

h. requiring oxygen

i. the cellular organelles responsible for producing ATP aerobically; made of membranes (lipid and protein) with enzymes mounted on them

j. the pathway in which glucose is metabolized to lactate (by anaerobic glycolysis) in the muscle, lactate travels to the liver where it is converted back to glucose, and then glucose returns to the muscle

18. _____ anabolism

19. _____ catabolism

20. _____ fatty acid oxidation

21. _____ gluconeogenesis

22. _____ keto acids

23. _____ ketone bodies

24. _____ oxaloacetate

25. _____ metabolism

a. a carbohydrate intermediate of the TCA cycle

b. reactions in which small molecules are put together to build larger ones, requiring energy

d. the metabolic breakdown of fatty acids to acetyl CoA

c. compounds produced during the incomplete breakdown of fat when glucose is not available

e. organic acids that contain a carbonyl group (C=O)

f. the sum total of all the chemical reactions that go on in living cells

g. making glucose from noncarbohydrate sources such as amino acids or glycerol

h. reactions in which large molecules are broken down to smaller ones, releasing energy

Sample Test Questions

Select the best answer for each question.

1. Photosynthesis is:
   a. the sum total of chemical reactions.
   b. a reaction that releases energy.
   c. the production of fuel for the body in the liver.
   d. the process of plants making simple sugars.

2. Compounds that the body can use for energy are called:
   a. fuels.
   b. vitamins.
   c. minerals.
   d. enzymes.

3. Energy, water, and carbon dioxide are released during what process?
   a. Photosynthesis
   b. Metabolism
   c. Anabolism
   d. Energy storage

4. Nutrients that are oxidized in the body to yield energy are:
   a. water, carbohydrate, fat, protein, vitamins, and minerals.
   b. carbohydrate, fat, protein, vitamins, and minerals.
   c. carbohydrate, fat, protein, and vitamins.
   d. carbohydrate, fat, and protein.
   e. carbohydrate and vitamins.

5. Reactions in which compounds are broken down into simpler molecules are called _____ reactions.
   a. anabolic
   b. catabolic
   c. gluconeogenic
   d. ergogenic

6. Complex organic molecules that work to facilitate the activity of enzymes are:
   a. adenosines.
   b. phosphates.
   c. coenzymes.
   d. hormones.

7. Which of the following statements is **false** regarding coupled reactions?
   a. Coupled reactions do not include the hydrolysis of ATP.
   b. Coupled reactions include the use of ATP during catabolism to power an anabolic reaction.
   c. Coupled reactions involve a transfer of energy.
   d. Coupled reactions have been referred to as a metabolic duet.

8. A three-carbon compound reversibly convertible to glucose is:
   a. an amino acid.
   b. pyruvate.
   c. acetyl CoA.
   d. a fatty acid.
   e. glucose.

9. When glucose is split in half, it yields two molecules of:
   a. acetate.
   b. glycerol.
   c. pyruvate.
   d. water.
   e. monosaccharides.

10. What part(s) of a triglyceride molecule can be made into glucose?
    a. Short-chain fatty acids
    b. Medium-chain fatty acids
    c. Long-chain fatty acids
    d. All fatty acids
    e. Glycerol

11. The process of glucose being split is called:
    a. the electron transport chain.
    b. the TCA cycle.
    c. gluconeogenesis.
    d. glycolysis.

12. Pyruvate is converted to lactate in:
    a. an anaerobic pathway.
    b. an aerobic pathway.
    c. pyruvate oxidation.
    d. glycolysis.

13. The concentration of lactate increases dramatically after:
    a. aerobic exercise.
    b. high-intensity exercise.
    c. low-intensity exercise.
    d. rest.

14. If the cells need energy and oxygen is available:
    a. lactate builds up.
    b. the Cori cycle is activated.
    c. pyruvate molecules enter the mitochondria.
    d. anaerobic metabolism begins.

15. When fatty acids are metabolized to yield energy, this is called:
    a. oxidation.
    b. glycolysis.
    c. deamination.
    d. ketosis.

16. The reaction which removes the NH$_2$ group from an amino acid is called:
    a. transamination.
    b. deamination.
    c. nitrogenation.
    d. hydrogenation.

17. Nitrogen from amino groups is excreted from the body in:
    a. urea.
    b. ammonia.
    c. nitrogen gas.
    d. amino acids.

18. Which of the following is **false** about the TCA cycle?
    a. It regenerates acetyl CoA.
    b. It requires oxaloacetate in the first and last steps.
    c. It requires ample carbohydrate.
    d. Each turn of the TCA cycle releases 8 electrons.

19. Which of the following is **false** about the electron transport chain?
    a. It is the final pathway in energy nutrient catabolism.
    b. It results in release of ATP to the cytoplasm.
    c. It consists of proteins that serve as carriers.
    d. The carriers are on the inner membrane of the nucleus.

20. When glucose is consumed in excess of body needs, the excess glucose is:
    a. not absorbed from the small intestine.
    b. excreted in the feces.
    c. stored as glucose.
    d. stored as glycogen only.
    e. stored as glycogen and fat.

21. Energy is stored in the body for future use as:
    a. triglycerides.
    b. glycerol.
    c. cholesterol.
    d. lecithin.

22. Which of the following statements is **true** regarding feasting?
    a. The storage form of energy depends on the type of energy-yielding nutrient consumed.
    b. Food energy excess cannot be stored in the body.
    c. Excess carbohydrate and fat are the only nutrients that can make you fat.
    d. Excess protein can be stored as fat.

23. Which of the following statements is **false** regarding fasting?
    a. Glucose is the preferred fuel for cells of the brain and nervous system.
    b. During fasting, body protein stores break down.
    c. During fasting, ketone bodies are produced.
    d. During fasting, fat cannot be used for energy.

24. During the second phase of fasting the body adapts by producing what alternative energy source?
    a. Glycogen
    b. Ammonia
    c. Pyruvate
    d. Ketone bodies

25. The condition of elevated urine ketones is called:
    a. ketonemia.
    b. ketosis.
    c. ketonuria.
    d. acidosis.

26. Which of the following is **false** regarding ketosis?
    a. It induces a loss of appetite.
    b. It causes acetone breath.
    c. It increases metabolism.
    d. It causes the pH of the blood to drop.

27. Short-term fasting usually produces:
    a. rapid weight loss.
    b. rapid fat loss.
    c. lean tissue gains.
    d. All of the above

92

28. Symptoms of starvation include all of the following **except**:
    a. wasting.
    b. accelerated metabolism.
    c. lowered body temperature.
    d. reduced resistance to disease.

29. Psychological effects of food deprivation include:
    a. muscle wasting, slowed heart rate, and depression.
    b. significant loss of body fat, loss of water, and anxiety.
    c. significant loss of body weight, hunger, and elation.
    d. depression, anxiety, and food-related dreams.

30. Which of the following statements is **false** regarding starvation?
    a. It slows energy output.
    b. Its progression differs among a starving child, an adult fasting for religious reasons, and the person with anorexia.
    c. It is physically and emotionally hazardous.
    d. It increases the breakdown of fat.

Short Answer Questions

1. Two types of reactions are:

    a. building: _____   b. breakdown: _____

2. Two helpers in metabolic reactions are:

    a.   b.

3. The energy nutrients are broken down into these basic units:

    a. carbohydrate: _____   c. protein: _____

    b. lipids: _____

4. How many carbons is in each of these compounds?

    a. glucose: _____   d. amino acids: _____

    b. glycerol: _____   e. pyruvate: _____

    c. fatty acids: _____   f. acetyl CoA: _____

5. The body can convert glycerol to:

    a.   b.

6. The body requires glucose for:

    a.   b.

7. Amino acids can enter the energy pathways in these ways:

    a.   c.

    b.

8. These energy-yielding nutrients yield glucose:

    a.   c.

    b.

9. These energy-yielding nutrients can be used to manufacture nonessential amino acids:

   a.   c.

   b.

10. Adaptations to fasting include:

    a.   c.

    b.

11. Weight loss as a result of ketosis reflects loss of:

    a.   c.

    b.   d.

Problem Solving

1. If Oliver, a healthy adult, meets his energy needs for the day with his food intake but also drinks a soda that provides 41 g of carbohydrate (in excess of his needs), how much energy will his body store (in kcal)?

2. Assuming that 1 ounce of body fat is equivalent to 219 kcal, how much fat will Oliver's body store using the energy from his soda?

3. If Oliver had consumed the same amount of excess energy as provided by the soda in the form of lipids instead of carbohydrates, would this affect the amount of energy stored in his body? If so, how?

Figure Identification

Identify the following structures, pathways, or processes.

1.

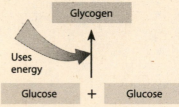 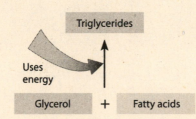 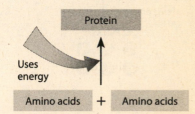

94

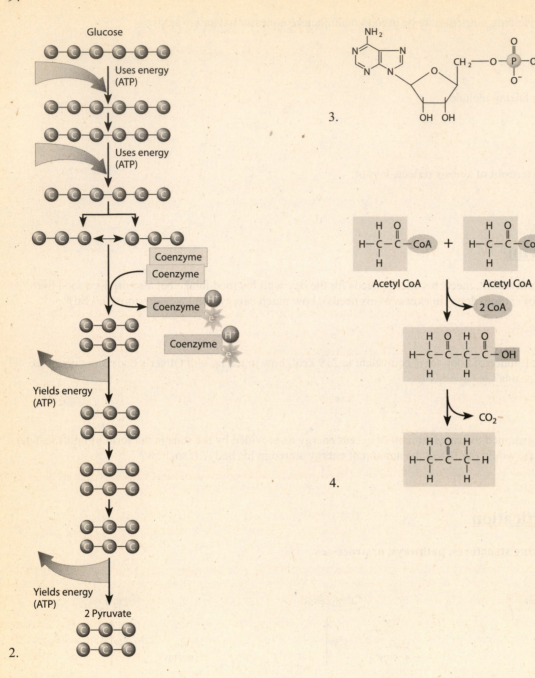

Glucose

Uses energy
(ATP)

Uses energy
(ATP)

Coenzyme

Coenzyme

Coenzyme

Coenzyme

Yields energy
(ATP)

Yields energy
(ATP)

2 Pyruvate

2.

3.

4.

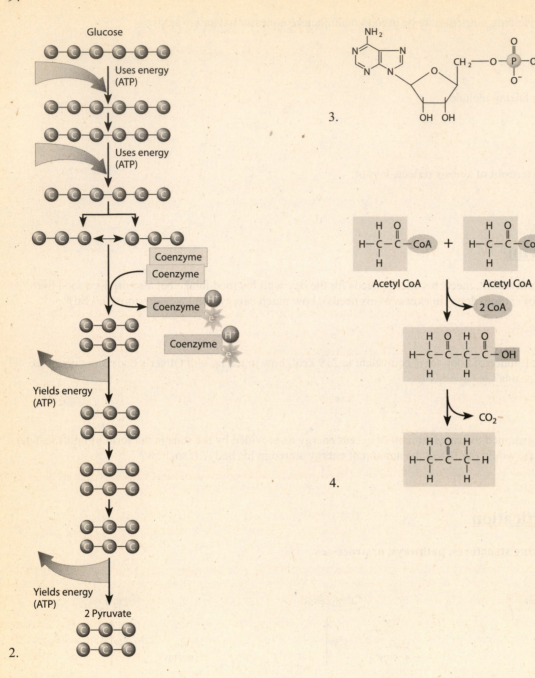

H_3C

$H \quad O$

$H-C-C-CoA$

H

Acetyl CoA

$+$

$H \quad O$

$H-C-C-CoA$

H

Acetyl CoA

$+$

H_2O

2 CoA

$H \quad O \quad H \quad O$

$H-C-C-C-C-OH$

$H \quad H$

CO_2

$H \quad O \quad H$

$H-C-C-C-H$

$H \quad H$

❧ Chapter 7 Answer Key ❧

Summing Up

1. glucose
2. amino
3. coenzymes
4. anabolism
5. catabolism
6. ATP
7. anabolism
8. glycolysis
9. pyruvate
10. lactate
11. acetyl CoA
12. irreversible
13. glucose
14. pyruvate
15. glycerol
16. fatty acids
17. TCA
18. fat
19. glucose
20. fat
21. nitrogen
22. deamination
23. acetyl CoA
24. electron
25. hundreds
26. enzyme
27. exceeds
28. protein
29. efficient
30. adaptations
31. energy
32. glycerol
33. ketones
34. metabolism
35. energy
36. metabolism.

Chapter Study Questions

1. Metabolism includes all chemical reactions, both anabolic and catabolic, that occur in living cells; for example, starch is metabolized to glucose. Anabolic reactions put small molecules together to build larger ones; for example, glycerol + fatty acids = triglyceride. Catabolic reactions break down large molecules to smaller ones; for example, triglyceride = glycerol + fatty acids.

2. ATP (adenosine triphosphate) is used as energy currency in metabolic reactions. This molecule includes adenosine plus 3 phosphate groups linked by high-energy bonds. When ATP is formed from ADP (adenosine diphosphate) by attaching a phosphate group, energy is stored within one of these high-energy bonds. The energy can then be released when needed by breaking off the third phosphate group and converting ATP back to ADP.

3. Coenzymes are complex organic molecules that work with enzymes to facilitate the enzymes' activity; they enable enzymes to do their work.

4. Glucose, glycerol, fatty acids, and amino acids. Glucose has 6 carbons, glycerol has 3 carbons, fatty acids usually have multiples of 2 carbons (commonly 16 or 18), and amino acids have 2, 3, or more carbons.

5. Aerobic metabolism refers to chemical reactions that require oxygen; anaerobic reactions do not require oxygen. Insufficient oxygen favors anaerobic metabolism, which relies on glucose as the primary fuel and results in lactate production.

6. When nitrogen is stripped from amino acids (deamination), ammonia is produced. The liver detoxifies ammonia before releasing it into the bloodstream by combining it with another waste product, carbon dioxide, to produce urea (see Chapter 6). Urea is filtered out of the blood by the kidneys and then excreted in urine.

7. Glucose to pyruvate to acetyl CoA to carbon dioxide. Glycerol to pyruvate either to glucose or to acetyl CoA to carbon dioxide. Fatty acids to acetyl CoA to carbon dioxide. Protein can be broken down to amino acids, and if used for energy, it must be deaminated (its nitrogen-containing amino group must be removed). Some amino acids can be used to make pyruvate and others can be used to make acetyl CoA.

8. Each can be broken down to pyruvate and/or acetyl CoA, which can be built up into fat. Dietary triglycerides can be simply broken down to glycerol and fatty acids and then reassembled as triglycerides within cells.

9. The body first draws on carbohydrate (glycogen) and fat reserves. When glycogen reserves are exhausted, body protein is used to make glucose; as the fast continues, ketones are made to meet energy needs of the nervous system, sparing protein. The body slows its metabolism, reducing its energy output and fat loss. Ketone bodies are compounds produced during the incomplete breakdown of fat when glucose is not available. Ketosis is the buildup of ketone bodies in the blood and urine.

10. Weight loss represents a loss of glycogen, protein, water, and minerals, not just a loss of fat. Both lean tissues and fat stores are catabolized when energy intake is less than needs. During either fasting or carbohydrate restriction severe enough to induce ketosis, the body adapts by utilizing more ketones derived from fats for energy. However, before this occurs, glycogen, muscle proteins, and the water that was associated with them

are lost (as weight loss) as the body undergoes gluconeogenesis in response to the low availability of carbohydrate. Fat losses on ketogenic diets are no greater than on other kcal-restricted diets.

Key Terms Practice

1. lactate
2. pyruvate
3. CoA
4. enzymes
5. coenzymes
6. glycolysis
7. fuel
8. d
9. h
10. g
11. b
12. j
13. c
14. f
15. i
16. a
17. e
18. b
19. h
20. d
21. g
22. e
23. c
24. a
25. f

Sample Test Questions

1. d (p. 197)
2. a (pp. 197-198)
3. b (p. 198)
4. d (p. 199)
5. b (p. 199)
6. c (p. 200)
7. a (p. 199)
8. b (pp. 202, 205)
9. c (p. 203)
10. e (p. 207)
11. d (p. 203)
12. a (p. 205)
13. b (pp. 205-206)
14. c (p. 206)
15. a (p. 207)
16. b (p. 207)
17. a (p. 207)
18. a (pp. 210-212)
19. d (p. 212)
20. e (pp. 213-214)
21. a (pp. 213, 216)
22. d (pp. 213-215)
23. d (pp. 215-217)
24. d (p. 217)
25. c (p. 217)
26. c (pp. 217-218)
27. a (p. 218)
28. b (p. 218)
29. d (p. 218)
30. b (p. 218)

Short Answer Questions

1. a. anabolism; b. catabolism
2. enzymes, coenzymes
3. a. glucose; b. glycerol + fatty acids; c. amino acids
4. a. 6; b. 3; c. multiples of 2; d. 2 or 3 or more; e. 3; f. 2
5. glucose, pyruvate
6. red blood cells, nervous system
7. converted to pyruvate; converted to acetyl CoA; enter the TCA cycle directly
8. carbohydrates, glycerol part of lipid, protein
9. carbohydrates, glycerol part of lipid, protein
10. making glucose (gluconeogenesis), making ketone bodies, conserving energy
11. glycogen, protein, body fluids, minerals

Problem Solving

1. 41 g × 4 kcal/g = 164 kcal. Storing carbohydrate as body fat requires 25% of the ingested energy intake, so only 75% of the kcal are stored. 0.75 × 164 kcal = 125 kcal.

2. 123 kcal divided by 219 kcal per oz. of fat = 0.56 oz.

3. Yes; since storing dietary lipid as body fat requires only 5% of ingested energy, more (95%) of the kcal will be stored as fat. 0.95 × 164 kcal = 156 kcal or 0.71 oz. of fat.

Figure Identification

1. anabolic reactions
2. glycolysis
3. ATP
4. ketone body formation

✆ Chapter 8 ~ Energy Balance and Body Composition ✆

Chapter Outline

I. Energy Balance
II. Energy In: The kCalories Foods Provide
   A. Food Composition
   B. Food Intake
     1. Hunger
     2. Satiation
     3. Satiety
     4. Overriding Hunger and Satiety
     5. Sustaining Satiation and Satiety
     6. Message Central—The Hypothalamus
III. Energy Out: The kCalories the Body Expends
   A. Components of Energy Expenditure
     1. Basal Metabolism
     2. Physical Activity
     3. Thermic Effect of Food
     4. Adaptive Thermogenesis
   B. Estimating Energy Requirements
IV. Body Weight and Body Composition
   A. Defining Healthy Body Weight
     1. The Criterion of Fashion
     2. The Criterion of Health
     3. Body Mass Index
   B. Body Fat and Its Distribution
     1. Some People Need Less Body Fat
     2. Some People Need More Body Fat
     3. Fat Distribution
     4. Waist Circumference
     5. Other Measures of Body Composition
V. Health Risks Associated with Body Weight and Body Fat
   A. Health Risks of Underweight
   B. Health Risks of Overweight
     1. Cardiovascular Disease
     2. Type 2 Diabetes
     3. Inflammation and the Metabolic Syndrome
     4. Cancer
   C. Fit and Fat versus Sedentary and Slim
VI. Eating Disorders
   A. The Female Athlete Triad
     1. Disordered Eating
     2. Amenorrhea
     3. Osteoporosis
   B. Other Dangerous Practices of Athletes
   C. Preventing Eating Disorders in Athletes
   D. Anorexia Nervosa
     1. Characteristics of Anorexia Nervosa
     2. Treatment of Anorexia Nervosa
   E. Bulimia Nervosa
     1. Characteristics of Bulimia Nervosa
     2. Treatment of Bulimia Nervosa
   F. Binge-Eating Disorder
   G. Eating Disorders in Society

Summing Up

When energy consumed equals energy 1._____, a person is in energy 2._____ and body weight is stable. If more energy is taken in than is expended, a person 3._____ weight. If more energy is expended than is taken in, a person 4._____ weight.

A mixture of signals governs a person's 5._____ behaviors. Hunger and 6._____ initiate eating, whereas 7._____ and satiety stop and delay eating, respectively. Each responds to messages from the 8._____ and hormonal systems. Superimposed on these signals are complex factors involving 9._____, habits, and other aspects of human behavior.

A person in energy 10._____ takes in energy from food and expends much of it on 11._____ metabolic activities, some of it on physical activities, and a little on the 12._____ _____ of food. Energy requirements 13._____ from person to person, depending on such factors as gender, age, weight, and 14._____ as well as the intensity and 15._____ of physical activity. All of these factors must be considered when estimating energy requirements.

The body mass index (BMI) is based on 16._____ in kilograms (kg) relative to 17._____ in meters (m) squared. As a useful measure of a person's weight status, the BMI serves as a reliable indicator of

98

18._____ disease risks, but it says little about body 19._____. The ideal amount of body fat varies from person to person, but researchers have found that body fat in excess of 20.____ percent for young men and 21.____ percent for young women (the levels rise slightly with age) poses health risks.

22._____ obesity is measured by 23._____ circumference and indicates excess abdominal fat distributed around the trunk of the body. Central obesity contributes to 24._____ diseases, but whether those risks are greater than fat elsewhere in the body is uncertain.

The weight appropriate for an individual depends largely on factors specific to that individual, including body fat 25._____, family health history, and current 26._____ status. At the extremes, both overweight and 27._____ carry clear risks to health.

Chapter Study Questions

1. What are the consequences of an unbalanced energy budget?

2. Define *hunger*, *appetite*, *satiation*, and *satiety* and describe how each influences food intake.

3. Describe the extent to which foods produce satiation and sustain satiety.

4. Describe each component of energy expenditure. What factors influence each? How can energy expenditure be estimated?

5. Describe factors that affect the BMR.

6. Distinguish between body weight and body composition. What assessment techniques are used to measure each?

7. What problems are involved in defining "ideal" body weight?

8. What is central obesity and what is its relationship to disease?

9. What are risks of underweight?

10. What risks are associated with excess body weight and excess body fat?

Key Terms Practice

To complete the crossword puzzle, identify the key term that best matches each definition.

Across:
1. The feeling of fullness and satisfaction that occurs after a meal and inhibits eating until the next meal.
3. Too much body fat with adverse health effects; BMI 30 or higher.
6. Having the power to suppress hunger and inhibit eating.
8. Body weight greater than the weight range that is considered healthy; BMI 25 to 29.9.
9. The painful sensation caused by a lack of food that initiates food-seeking behavior.
10. An immunological response to cellular injury characterized by an increase in white blood cells.

Down:
2. The generation of heat; used in physiology and nutrition studies as an index of how much energy the body is expending.
4. The feeling of satisfaction and fullness that occurs during a meal and halts eating.
5. Body weight lower than the weight range that is considered healthy; BMI below 18.5.
7. The integrated response to the sight, smell, thought, or taste of food that initiates or delays eating.

Match the key terms with their definitions.

11. _____ basal metabolic rate
12. _____ basal metabolism
13. _____ bomb calorimeter
14. _____ energy balance
15. _____ hypothalamus
16. _____ lean body mass
17. _____ neuropeptide Y
18. _____ physiological fuel value
19. _____ resting metabolic rate

a. the kcalories consumed from foods and beverages compared with the energy expended through metabolic processes and physical activities
b. an instrument that measures the heat energy released when foods are burned, thus providing an estimate of the potential energy of the foods
c. the number of kcalories that the body derives from a food
d. a brain center that controls activities such as maintenance of water balance, regulation of body temperature, and control of appetite
e. a chemical produced in the brain that stimulates appetite, diminishes energy expenditure, and increases fat storage
f. the body minus its fat
g. the rate of energy use for metabolism under specified conditions: after a 12-hour fast and restful sleep, without any physical activity or emotional excitement, and in a comfortable setting
h. a measure of the energy use of a person at rest in a comfortable setting, but with less stringent criteria for recent food intake and physical activity
i. the energy needed to maintain life when a body is at complete digestive, physical, and emotional rest

20. _____ adaptive thermogenesis
21. _____ body composition
22. _____ body mass index
23. _____ central obesity
24. _____ insulin resistance
25. _____ subcutaneous fat
26. _____ thermic effect of food
27. _____ visceral fat
28. _____ waist circumference

a. an estimation of the energy required to process food (digest, absorb, transport, metabolize, and store ingested nutrients)
b. adjustments in energy expenditure related to changes in environment such as extreme cold and to physiological events such as overfeeding, trauma, and changes in hormone status
c. excess fat around the trunk of the body
d. a measure of a person's weight relative to height; determined by dividing the weight (in kilograms) by the square of the height (in meters)
e. fat stored within the abdominal cavity in association with the internal abdominal organs
f. the proportions of muscle, bone, fat, and other tissue that make up a person's total body weight
g. fat stored directly under the skin
h. an anthropometric measurement used to assess a person's abdominal fat
i. the condition in which a normal amount of insulin produces a subnormal effect in muscle, adipose, and liver cells, resulting in an elevated fasting glucose

Sample Test Questions

Select the best answer for each question.

1. For each _____ kcal eaten in excess, one pound of body fat is stored.
   a. 2,000
   b. 2,500
   c. 3,000
   d. 3,500

2. An instrument that measures the heat energy released when foods are burned is a(n):
   a. body mass index.
   b. indirect calorimeter.
   c. bomb calorimeter.
   d. heat food release mechanism.

3. The feeling of fullness that occurs during a meal and halts eating is called:
   a. satiation.
   b. satiety.
   c. purging.
   d. appetite.

4. If something has the power to suppress hunger and inhibit eating, you describe it as:
   a. appetite control.
   b. high in energy density.
   c. satiating.
   d. satiation.

5. Which of the following statements is **true** about resting metabolic rate?
   a. It is slightly lower than the BMR.
   b. It is lower than the thermic effect of food.
   c. It is the same as diet-induced thermogenesis.
   d. It is a measure of energy use of a person at rest in a comfortable setting.

6. Which of the following describes the process of thermogenesis?
   a. Burning of fat
   b. Synthesis of fat
   c. Generation of heat
   d. Generation of water

7. What method is used to measure the amount of heat given off by the body?
   a. Bomb calorimetry
   b. Basal calorimetry
   c. Direct calorimetry
   d. Indirect calorimetry

8. Additional energy that is spent when a person must adapt to extremely cold conditions is called:
   a. basal metabolism.
   b. resting metabolism.
   c. adaptive thermogenesis.
   d. rebound thermogenesis.

9. The number of kcalories that the body derives from a food is:
   a. called the physiological fuel value.
   b. called the calorimetry value.
   c. greater than the number of kcalories measured by direct calorimetry.
   d. less precise than computing values based on grams of energy-yielding nutrients.

10. The amount of energy a food provides may be measured by burning the food and measuring the:
    a. vitamins produced.
    b. heat released.
    c. water produced.
    d. water released.
    e. weight of the ash remaining.

11. The energy used by the body completely at rest after a 12-hour fast is:
    a. specific dynamic energy.
    b. basal metabolism.
    c. active energy.
    d. total kcalories expended.
    e. zero energy.

12. Which of the following will reduce BMR?
   a. Fever
   b. Fasting
   c. Nicotine
   d. High thyroid activity

13. In general, _____ have a lower BMR than _____.
   a. adolescents, adults
   b. large people, smaller people
   c. younger adults, older adults
   d. women, men

14. What is the major factor that determines metabolic rate?
   a. Age
   b. Gender
   c. Amount of fat tissue
   d. Amount of lean body mass

15. Which of the following increases the metabolic rate?
   a. Fever
   b. Fasting
   c. Inactivity
   d. Malnutrition

16. Which of the following statements is **true** regarding satiation?
   a. It is best achieved by high simple carbohydrate intake.
   b. Fat has a weak effect on satiation.
   c. Protein is the most satiating.
   d. Satiation is not influenced by energy-yielding nutrients.

17. Which chemical causes carbohydrate cravings?
   a. Thyroxin
   b. Neuropeptide Y
   c. Estrogen
   d. Cholecystokinin

18. Which method provides a precise measurement of bone tissue, fat mass, and fat distribution in all but extremely obese subjects?
   a. Dual energy X-ray absorptiometry
   b. Skinfold measures
   c. Hydrodensitometry
   d. Bioelectrical impedance

19. A BMI of 27 is considered:
   a. underweight.
   b. normal.
   c. overweight.
   d. obese.

20. If you eat 2,400 kcalories a day, about _____ will be used for the thermic effect of food.
   a. 24 kcalories
   b. 240 kcalories
   c. 100 kcalories
   d. 10 kcalories
   e. 3,500 kcalories

21. Which of the following methods most accurately assesses body fatness?
   a. Skinfold measurements
   b. The accepted style of the culture
   c. Undressing and standing before a mirror to see how you look to yourself
   d. The fit of your clothes
   e. Comparing weight with standard weight charts

22. Which of the following statements is **true**?
   a. Fashion is helpful when assessing ideal body weights.
   b. Fashion has contributed to establishing healthy standards for body weight.
   c. Perceived body size is almost identical to actual body size.
   d. Fashion presents unrealistic and unhealthy ideals for body size.

23. An index of a person's weight in relation to height is called:
   a. body mass index.
   b. height-to-weight index.
   c. ideal body weight index.
   d. desirable body weight index.

24. Which of the following statements is **false** about the body mass index?
    a. It reflects height and weight measures.
    b. It does not reflect body composition.
    c. It is ideal for estimating health risk in all populations.
    d. It may misclassify muscular athletes as overweight or obese.

25. Which measures of waist circumferences for women and men indicate health risk?
    a. 22 or more inches for women and 25 or more inches for men
    b. 25 or more inches for women and 30 or more inches for men
    c. 30 or more inches for women and 35 or more inches for men
    d. 35 or more inches for women and 40 or more inches for men

26. Which statement is **true** regarding the correlation between BMI and disease risk?
    a. It suggests a greater likelihood of shortened life expectancy for those with high BMIs.
    b. It reveals the causes of disease.
    c. High BMI is not correlated with chronic disease risk.
    d. BMI provides information about life expectancy with 99 percent accuracy.

27. Underweight people may be at risk for:
    a. malnutrition.
    b. infertility.
    c. lean tissue loss if they develop cancer.
    d. All of the above

28. Obese persons are faced with:
    1. a risk of earlier death due to a host of physical problems.
    2. the likely precipitation of type 2 diabetes.
    3. a lowered accident rate due to the protection from adipose tissue.
    4. an increased risk of cardiovascular disease.
    5. greater economic success because of higher job productivity.

    a. 1, 3, 5
    b. 1, 2, 4
    c. 1, 2, 5
    d. 2, 3, 4
    e. 3, 4, 5

29. Central-body fat cells seem to be _____ than lower-body fat cells.
    a. less likely to promote type 2 diabetes
    b. more responsive to insulin
    c. more insulin resistant
    d. smaller

30. Accumulation of fat and activation of genes that code for proteins involved in inflammation causes:
    a. obesity.
    b. diabetes.
    c. metabolic syndrome.
    d. insulin resistance.

Short Answer Questions

1. Components of weight gained or lost rapidly include:

    a.   c.

    b.

2. Two factors that may initiate eating are:

    a.   b.

3. Two factors that inhibit eating are:

    a. during a meal: _____   b. after a meal: _____

4. Four components of energy expenditure are:

   a.   c.

   b.   d.

5. Factors that increase BMR include:

   a.   g.

   b.   h.

   c.   i.

   d.   j.

   e.   k.

   f.

6. Fat's roles in the body include:

   a.

   b.

   c.

   d.

   e.

7. Terms used to refer to fat that is stored around the organs of the abdomen include:

   a.   c.

   b.   d.

8. BMI ranges for healthy weight, overweight, and obesity are:

   a. healthy weight: _____   c. obesity: _____

   b. overweight: _____

9. Cardiovascular disease risk factors associated with obesity include:

   a.   c.

   b.   d.

Problem Solving

1. Estimate the energy required for basal metabolism for a 175-pound man for a 24-hour period.

2. A person's EER is 2500 kcalories per day. This person wants to lose 1 pound of fat a week. How many kcalories should the person consume each day?

3. A person's body weight is 150 pounds and this person is 75 inches tall. Calculate the BMI.

4. A person's body weight is 132 pounds and this person is 5 feet 6 inches tall. Calculate the BMI.

5. A person's EER is 3000 kcalories per day. If 65% is BMR, 10% is thermic effect of food, and 25% is physical activities, how many kcalories is this person expending in each component of energy expenditure?

6. A person has a BMI of 26 and is 5'8". She desires to have a BMI of 24. Calculate her desired body weight.

7. Calculate how much energy a 150-pound person would expend doing 30 minutes of vigorous aerobic dance.

8. Calculate how much energy a 170-pound person would expend running for 20 minutes at 9 mph.

9. Compute the daily energy needs for a woman, age 47, who is 5 feet 6 inches tall, weighs 130 lbs., and is lightly active.

10. Compute the daily energy needs for a man, age 21, who is 5 feet 10 inches tall, weighs 142 lbs., and is active.

⟲ Chapter 8 Answer Key ⟲

Summing Up

1. expended
2. balance
3. gains
4. loses
5. eating
6. appetite
7. satiation
8. nervous
9. emotions
10. balance
11. basal
12. thermic effect
13. vary
14. height
15. duration
16. weight
17. height
18. chronic
19. composition
20. 22
21. 27
22. Central
23. waist
24. chronic
25. distribution
26. health
27. underweight.

Chapter Study Questions

1. Weight gain, and possibly overfatness, can result from positive energy balance and weight loss, and possibly underweight, can result from negative energy balance.

2. Hunger is the painful sensation caused by the physiological need for food that initiates food seeking and eating; appetite is the integrated response to the sight, smell, thought, or taste of food that initiates or delays eating. Satiation is the feeling of satisfaction and fullness that occurs during a meal and halts eating; satiety is a feeling of fullness after a meal that inhibits eating until the next meal. Hunger and appetite are likely to increase food intake, though sometimes appetite may decrease it. Satiation determines how much food is consumed during a meal. Satiety determines how much time passes between meals. A high level of satiety is likely to decrease food intake between meals.

3. This partially depends on the nutrient composition of a meal. Protein is considered the most satiating. Too little protein can leave a person feeling hungry, whereas including protein at a meal provides satiety and decreases energy intake at the next meal. Fructose in a sugary drink seems to stimulate appetite and increase food intake. High-fiber foods of low energy density provide satiation by filling the stomach and delaying nutrient absorption. High-fat foods (which are typically energy dense and lower in volume) provide little satiation during a meal but contribute to satiety once they reach the intestine.

4. Basal metabolism: energy needed to maintain life when a body is at complete rest; influenced by lean body mass, health and nutrition status, and many other factors (see Table 8-1). Physical activity: voluntary movement of the skeletal muscles and support systems; influenced by the individual's lifestyle. Thermic effect of food: energy required to process food; influenced by macronutrient composition of the diet. Adaptive thermogenesis (not when calculating energy requirements): energy expended in response to dramatic changes in circumstances within the body, such as stress; influenced by ambient temperature, nutritional status, and medical conditions such as trauma. Energy expenditure can be estimated using predictive equations or indirect calorimetry. (See the How to Estimate Energy Requirements box for specific equations.)

5. Age—lean mass diminishes with age, slowing the BMR; tall people have high BMR than short people; growth stages increase BMR; people with greater lean body mass (typically males) have a higher BMR than those with less lean tissue (typically females); fever raises BMR; stresses such as disease increase BMR; heat and cold changes in the environment raise BMR; fasting, starvation, and malnutrition lower BMR; some hormones can increase or decrease BMR; smoking and caffeine increase energy expenditure; BMR is reduced during sleep.

6. Weight depends on frame size, lean mass, fat mass, and bone weight; body composition is more important than weight but is difficult to measure. Location of body fat is more important than quantity of body fat; fat around the waist and abdomen poses a greater risk than fat in other areas. Weight is assessed by weighing the person using a scale. Body composition assessment techniques include: total body water, radioactive potassium count, near-infrared spectrophotometry, ultrasound, computer tomography, and magnetic resonance imaging.

7. Defining a healthy body weight is a complex issue. Our society sets unrealistic ideals for body weight, especially for women. These ideals usually impair the health of those who attempt to adhere to them. Body composition is another important issue. Two people may weigh the same but have different amounts of muscle and fat. The presence of more lean mass is beneficial. Another factor is the distribution of body fat. Fat stored within the abdomen (visceral fat) may pose a particular health risk. Finally, it may be advantageous for certain

individuals to have more or less body fat than the standard "ideal"; e.g., competitive endurance athletes who are very lean have a performance advantage.

8. Central obesity is excess fat within the abdomen and around the trunk of the body. Much research suggests that central obesity is an independent (from BMI) and significant risk factor for heart disease and mortality. Other studies, however, have found that obesity of any sort is the true risk factor, regardless of the location of fat.

9. An inability to preserve lean tissue during wasting diseases such as cancer or a digestive disorder, especially when it is accompanied by malnutrition; menstrual irregularities and infertility in underweight women; higher risk for giving birth to underweight babies; osteoporosis and bone fractures.

10. Increased risk of heart attacks, strokes, type 2 diabetes, high blood cholesterol, hypertension, sleep apnea, surgery complications, infertility, complications of pregnancy, certain types of cancer, osteoarthritis, gallbladder disease, kidney stones, respiratory problems, and disabilities.

Key Terms Practice

1. satiety	8. overweight	15. d	22. d
2. thermogenesis	9. hunger	16. f	23. c
3. obese	10. inflammation	17. e	24. i
4. satiation	11. g	18. c	25. g
5. underweight	12. i	19. h	26. a
6. satiating	13. b	20. b	27. e
7. appetite	14. a	21. f	28. h

Sample Test Questions

1. d (p. 232)	9. a (p. 232)	17. b (p. 236)	24. c (pp. 242-243)
2. c (p. 232)	10. b (p. 232)	18. a (p. 246)	25. d (pp. 244-245)
3. a (p. 233)	11. b (p. 236)	19. c (pp. 242, 243)	26. a (pp. 246-247)
4. c (p. 233)	12. b (p. 237)	20. b (p. 239)	27. d (p. 247)
5. d (p. 236)	13. d (p. 239)	21. a (pp. 241-242, 245-246)	28. b (pp. 247-248)
6. c (p. 236)	14. d (p. 237)	22. d (p. 241)	29. c (p. 248)
7. c (p. 236)	15. a (p. 237)	23. a (p. 242)	30. c (p. 248)
8. c (p. 239)	16. c (p. 235)		

Short Answer Questions

1. some fat, large amounts of fluid, some lean tissues such as muscle proteins and bone minerals

2. hunger, appetite

3. a. satiation; b. satiety

4. basal metabolism, physical activity, thermic effect of food, adaptive thermogenesis

5. younger age, greater height, growth, lean body composition, male gender, fever, stresses, environmental temperature, some hormones, smoking, caffeine

6. provides energy; insulates against temperature extremes; protects against physical shock; forms cell membranes; makes compounds such as hormones, vitamin D, and bile

7. visceral fat, intra-abdominal fat, central obesity, upper-body fat

8. a. 18.5-24.9; b. 25-29.9; c. 30 or greater

9. high LDL cholesterol, low HDL cholesterol, high blood pressure (hypertension), diabetes

Problem Solving

1. 175 lb. divided by 2.2 lb./kg = 79.5 kg
   79.5 kg × 24 kcal/kg/day = 1908 kcal/day

2. 3500 kcalories in a pound of fat divided by 7 days per week = 500
   2500 − 500 = 2000 kcalories per day

3. $(150 \div 75^2) \times 703 = (150 \div 5625) \times 703 = 18.7$

4. $(132 \div 66^2) \times 703 = 21.3$

5. 3000 × 0.65 = 1950 BMR kcalories per day
   3000 × 0.10 = 300 kcalories from thermic effect of food per day
   3000 × 0.25 = 750 physical activity kcalories per day

6. $24 = (\text{wt.} \div 68^2) \times 703$
   24 ÷ 703 = wt. ÷ 4624
   24 ÷ 703 × 4,624 = wt. = 158 lb.

7. Refer to Table 8-2 for kcal/lb./minute expended on various activities.
   150 lb. × 0.062 kcal/lb./min × 30 minutes = 9.3 kcal/min × 30 minutes = 279 kcalories

8. 170 lb. × 0.103 kcal/lb./min × 20 min = 17.51 kcal/min × 20 min = 350 kcalories

9. 130 lb. ÷ 2.2 lb./kg = 59 kg; 66 in. ÷ 39.37 in./m = 1.68 m
   EER = 354 − (6.91 × 47) + 1.12 × [(9.36 × 59) + (726 × 1.68)]
   EER = 354 − 325 + 1.12 × [552 + 1219]
   EER = 354 − 325 + 1.12 × 1771
   EER = 354 − 325 + 1983 = 2012 kcalories/day

10. 142 lb. ÷ 2.2 lb./kg = 65 kg; 70 in. ÷ 39.37 in./m = 1.8 m
    EER = 662 − (9.53 × 21) + 1.25 × [(15.91 × 65) + (539.6 × 1.8)]
    EER = 662 − 200 + 1.25 × [1034 + 971]
    EER = 462 + 1.25 × 2005 = 462 + 2506 = 2968 kcalories/day

Chapter 9 ~ Weight Management: Overweight, Obesity, and Underweight

Chapter Outline

I.   Overweight and Obesity
   A.   Fat Cell Development
   B.   Fat Cell Metabolism
   C.   Set-Point Theory
II. Causes of Overweight and Obesity
   A.   Genetics and Epigenetics
      1.   Leptin
      2.   Ghrelin
      3.   Uncoupling Proteins
   B.   Environment
      1.   Overeating
      2.   Physical Inactivity
III. Problems of Overweight and Obesity
   A.   Health Risks
      1.   Overweight in Good Health
      2.   Obese or Overweight with Risk Factors
      3.   Obese or Overweight with Life-Threatening Condition
   B.   Perceptions and Prejudices
      1.   Social Consequences
      2.   Psychological Problems
   C.   Dangerous Interventions
      1.   Fad Diets
      2.   Weight-Loss Products
      3.   Other Gimmicks
IV. Aggressive Treatments for Obesity
   A.   Drugs
   B.   Surgery
V.   Weight-Loss Strategies
   A.   Set Reasonable Goals
   B.   Eating Patterns
      1.   Be Realistic about Energy Intake
      2.   Emphasize Nutritional Adequacy
      3.   Eat Small Portions
      4.   Slow Down
      5.   Lower Energy Density
      6.   Remember Water
      7.   Focus on Fiber
      8.   Choose Fats Sensibly
      9.   Select Carbohydrates Carefully
      10. Watch for Other Empty kCalories

   C.   Physical Activity
      1.   Activity and Energy Expenditure
      2.   Activity and Discretionary kCalories
      3.   Activity and Metabolism
      4.   Activity and Body Composition
      5.   Activity and Appetite Control
      6.   Activity and Psychological Benefits
      7.   Choosing Activities
      8.   Spot Reducing
   D.   Environmental Influences
      1.   Atmosphere
      2.   Accessibility
      3.   Socializing
      4.   Distractions
      5.   Multiple Choices
      6.   Package and Portion Sizes
      7.   Serving Containers
   E.   Behavior and Attitude
      1.   Become Aware of Behaviors
      2.   Change Behaviors
      3.   Cognitive Skills
      4.   Personal Attitude
      5.   Support Groups
   F.   Weight Maintenance
   G.   Prevention
   H.   Community Programs
VI. Underweight
   A.   Problems of Underweight
   B.   Weight-Gain Strategies
      1.   Energy-Dense Foods
      2.   Regular Meals Daily
      3.   Large Portions
      4.   Extra Snacks
      5.   Juice and Milk
      6.   Exercising to Build Muscles
VII. The Latest and Greatest Weight-Loss Diet—Again
   A.   Fad Diets' Appeal
      1.   Don't Count kCalories
      2.   Follow a Plan
   B.   The Real Deal

Summing Up

Fat cells develop by increasing in 1._____ and size. Obesity prevention depends on maintaining a reasonable number of 2._____ cells. With weight gains or 3._____, the body adjusts in an attempt to return to its 4._____-_____ weight.

Obesity has many causes and most 5._____, creating a complex scenario.

6._____ factors, such as overeating and physical 7._____, may influence a person's genetic 8._____ to obesity.

The question of whether a person should lose weight depends on many 9._____: among them are the extent of 10._____, age, health, and 11._____ makeup. Not all obesity will cause 12._____ or shorten life expectancy. Just as there are unhealthy, normal-weight people, there are healthy,13._____ people. Some people may risk more in the process of losing weight than in remaining 14._____. Fad diets and weight-loss 15._____ can be as physically and psychologically damaging as excess body weight.

Overweight and 16._____ people may benefit most from improving eating and 17._____ habits. Those with high risks of medical problems may need more 18._____ treatment, including drugs or surgery. Such treatments may offer benefits, but also incur some 19._____.

A surefire remedy for obesity has yet to be found, although many people find a 20._____ of approaches to be most effective. Diet and exercise shift energy balance so that more energy is 21._____ than is taken in. Behavior 22._____ and cognitive 23._____ retrain habits to support a healthy eating and activity plan. Such a plan requires 24._____, individualization, and sometimes the assistance of a 25._____ _____ or support group.

Both the incidence of underweight and the health problems associated with it are less 26._____ than overweight and its associated problems. To gain weight, a person must train physically and 27._____ energy intake by selecting 28._____-_____ foods, eating regular meals, taking larger portions, and consuming extra snacks and beverages.

Chapter Study Questions

1. Discuss the prevalence of overweight and obesity in the United States.

2. Describe how the body's fat stores develop and suggest some reasons why it is difficult for an obese person to maintain weight loss.

3. What genetic factors contribute to obesity?

4.   What environmental factors contribute to obesity?

5.   Discuss some situations where weight loss is recommended and those where weight loss may not be recommended.

6.   Describe the perceptions and prejudices faced by overweight and obese people in our society.

7.   List several ineffective ways to treat obesity and explain why such methods are not recommended.

8.   Discuss some aggressive treatments for obesity.

9.   Discuss reasonable dietary strategies suitable for achieving and maintaining a healthy body weight.

10. What are the benefits of increased physical activity in a weight-loss program?

11. Describe the behavioral strategies recommended for losing weight and maintaining the desired weight.

12. Should an underweight person try to gain weight? Discuss the causes of underweight.

112

13. Describe strategies for weight gain.

Key Terms Practice

To complete the crossword puzzle, identify the key term that best matches each definition.

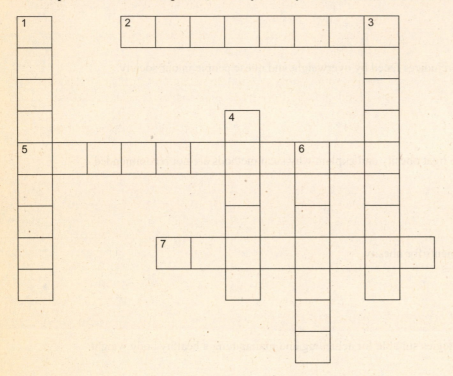

Across:

2. Popular eating plans that promise quick weight loss. Most severely limit certain foods or overemphasize others.
5. A body weight so low as to have adverse health effects; generally defined as BMI <18.5.
7. The appearance of a disease (usually infectious) or condition that attacks many people at the same time in the same region.

Down:

1. Supposedly, a lumpy form of fat; actually, a fraud.
3. A neurotransmitter important in sleep regulation, appetite control, and sensory perception, among other roles.
4. A protein produced by fat cells under direction of the *ob* gene that decreases appetite and increases energy expenditure.
6. A protein produced by the stomach cells that enhances appetite and decreases energy expenditure.

Match the key terms with their definitions.

8. _____ behavior modification

9. _____ brown adipose tissue

10. _____ clinically severe obesity

11. _____ gene pool

12. _____ lipoprotein lipase

13. _____ obesogenic environment

14. _____ set point

15. _____ successful weight-loss maintenance

16. _____ weight management

a. maintaining body weight in a healthy range by preventing gradual weight gains over time and losing weight if overweight, and by preventing weight losses and gaining weight if underweight

b. an enzyme that hydrolyzes triglycerides passing by in the bloodstream and directs their parts into the cells, where they can be metabolized or reassembled for storage

c. the point at which controls are set (for example, on a thermostat); name for the theory that proposes that the body tends to maintain a certain weight by means of its own internal controls

d. masses of specialized fat cells packed with pigmented mitochondria that produce heat instead of ATP

e. all the genetic information of a population at a given time

f. all the factors surrounding a person that promote weight gain, such as increased food intake, especially of unhealthy choices, and decreased physical activity

g. a BMI of 40 or greater or a BMI of 35 or greater with additional medical problems

h. the changing of behavior by the manipulation of antecedents (cues or environmental factors that trigger behavior), the behavior itself, and consequences (the penalties or rewards attached to behavior)

i. achieving a weight loss of at least 10% of initial body weight and maintaining the loss for at least one year

Sample Test Questions

Select the best answer for each question.

1. The prevalence of overweight and obesity in the U.S. continues to:
   a. decrease.
   b. remain high.
   c. remain low.
   d. rise and fall.

2. A person with a BMI of 26 is:
   a. underweight.
   b. at a healthy weight.
   c. overweight.
   d. obese.

3. Obesity is viewed as:
   a. a minor health risk.
   b. a condition that improves physical appearance.
   c. a problem only in developed countries.
   d. an epidemic.

4. Which statement about fat cell development is **true**?
   a. Obese people tend to have more fat cells.
   b. Enlarged fat cells inhibit cell proliferation.
   c. Weight loss results in a loss of fat cells.
   d. Fat is deposited only in adipose tissues.

5. How does lipoprotein lipase activity affect body fatness?
   a. It helps to regulate food intake and energy expenditure in response to fat stores.
   b. It promotes deposition and retention of fat around the hips and thighs in women.
   c. It reduces the likelihood of weight regain after weight loss.
   d. It decreases the efficiency of triglyceride removal from blood.

6. Which enzyme promotes efficient fat storage in both fat and muscle cells?
   a. Protease
   b. Brown fat lipase
   c. Leptin protease
   d. Lipoprotein lipase

7. The protein _____ is secreted by the stomach and promotes weight gain by stimulating appetite and promoting efficient fat storage.
   a. lipase
   b. leptin
   c. ghrelin
   d. insulin

8. _____ suggests that the body tends to maintain a certain weight by internal controls.
   a. LPL activity theory
   b. Cognitive restructuring theory
   c. Leptin theory
   d. Set-point theory

9. The obesity gene that codes for leptin is called the:
   a. *ob* gene.
   b. set point.
   c. *leptin* gene.
   d. *Gap* gene.

10. When leptin levels are high:
    a. it signals the hypothalamus.
    b. appetite is reduced.
    c. energy expenditure is slowed.
    d. a and b
    e. a, b, and c

11. Obese people typically experience which of the following?
    a. Prejudice in the workplace
    b. Negative stereotyping by acquaintances
    c. Embarrassment in social situations
    d. All of the above

12. Adverse reactions to fad diets can include:
    a. headaches and dizziness.
    b. nausea.
    c. death.
    d. a and b
    e. a, b, and c

13. What drug currently used to treat obesity suppresses appetite by enhancing the release of norepinephrine?
    a. Orlistat
    b. Benzocaine
    c. Phentermine
    d. Sibutramine

14. Uncoupling proteins:
    a. are inactive in brown fat.
    b. enhance development of obesity.
    c. cause resistance to weight gain.
    d. lower BMR.

15. A drug that inhibits fat absorption in the GI tract is:
    a. phentermine.
    b. orlistat.
    c. ephedrine.
    d. yohimbine.

16. Methods to induce weight loss by interfering with the amount of food consumed include all of the following **except**
    a. liposuction.
    b. gastric banding.
    c. reducing the size of the stomach.
    d. gastric bypass.

17. Which of the following does not describe the controversies involved in obesity treatment?
    a. Treating obesity is a simple task.
    b. Everyone cannot achieve thinness.
    c. Overweight people face discrimination.
    d. Self-esteem is harmed by repeated weight loss and gain.

18. Which of the following is a safe rate for weight loss?
    a. ½ to 2 pounds per week
    b. 3 to 5 pounds per week
    c. 10% of body weight over 2 months
    d. 15% of body weight over 3 months

19. What is the best approach to weight loss?
    a. Avoid foods containing carbohydrates.
    b. Reduce daily energy intake and increase energy expenditure.
    c. Eliminate all fats from the diet and decrease water intake.
    d. Greatly increase protein intake to prevent body protein loss.

20. To lose fat efficiently while retaining lean tissue, adults with a BMI between 27 and 35 need a deficit of _____ kcalories per day.
    a. 500
    b. 100
    c. 150
    d. 200

21. Fiber-rich foods usually offer:
    a. high energy density.
    b. large amounts of fat.
    c. high nutrient density.
    d. low satiety.

22. A benefit of the use of artificial sweeteners in a weight control program is:
    a. it lowers the energy density of food.
    b. it reduces hunger.
    c. it provides dramatic weight loss.
    d. a, b, and c

23. A helpful tip for weight loss is:
    a. Cut out all fats in the diet.
    b. Increase your daily energy intake.
    c. Avoid all foods containing carbohydrates.
    d. Increase your water intake.

24. Regular physical activity often results in all of the following **except**:
    a. lower energy expenditure.
    b. increased BMR.
    c. improved appetite control.
    d. stress reduction.

25. An average of at least _____ minutes of moderate-intensity activity per day is recommended for weight management.
    a. 30
    b. 45
    c. 60
    d. 90

26. Which of the following statements is **true** regarding exercise?
    a. Specific exercises can remove fat from certain targeted body parts.
    b. Exercise can assist in weight loss by burning fat.
    c. Exercise is only beneficial if it is done for 1 hour or more.
    d. Older people should not engage in physical activity.

27. To help maximize the long-term success of a person's weight-loss program, which of the following personal attitudes should be encouraged in the individual?
    a. Openness to examining emotional health status and whether stress triggers overeating
    b. Viewing the body realistically as being very fat rather than thin
    c. Refraining from expressing overconfidence in ability to lose weight
    d. Accepting that lack of exercising is a part of the lifestyle of most overweight people

28. All of the following are behavior modifications for losing weight **except**:
    a. shopping only when not hungry.
    b. tracking food consumption on a smart phone.
    c. exercising while watching television.
    d. eating food right out of the package.

29. Which of the following would probably not be part of a successful program of weight gain in an underweight individual?
    a. Engaging in physical exercise to build muscle tissue
    b. Consuming energy-dense foods
    c. Consuming energy-dense beverages
    d. Avoiding snacking between meals

30. Weight maintenance may require a person to expend as many as _____ kcalories per week through physical activities.
    a. 300   c. 3500
    b. 2500   d. 500

Short Answer Questions

1. The weight classifications based on BMI are:

    a.   c.

    b.   d.

2. Fat cells store excess triglycerides by increasing in:

    a.   b.

3. Hormones involved in appetite regulation include:

    a.   b.

4. Two major behavioral causes of obesity that are related to environmental factors are:

    a.   b.

5. Three indicators that health-care professionals use in evaluating the risks to health from obesity are:

    a.   c.

    b.

6. The factors that determine whether a person should lose weight include:

    a.   c.

    b.   d.

7. Aggressive treatments appropriate for obese people with high risks of medical problems include:

    a.   b.

8. Examples of behavioral strategies to support weight change include:

    a.

    b.

    c.

9. Benefits of physical activity in a weight-management program include:

   a.

   b.

   c.

   d.

   e.

   f.

   g.

10. Weight-gain strategies include:

    a.

    b.

    c.

    d.

    e.

    f.

Problem Solving

1. Calculate the energy density of a food item which weighs 75 grams and delivers 35 kcalories.

2. Calculate the energy density of a food item which weighs 60 grams and delivers 100 kcalories.

3. A person's EER is 4000 kcalories per day, current weight is 210 lb., and desired weight is 175 lb. This person plans to lose 1 pound of fat a week. How many kcalories should be consumed daily and (if the person is compliant) how long will it take to achieve the desired weight?

4. A creamy, mixed alcoholic beverage contains 2 grams of alcohol, 60 grams of carbohydrate, 20 grams of protein, and 40 grams of fat. Calculate the kcalories that this beverage can deliver. Would this beverage be an appropriate snack for someone on a weight-loss diet?

118

5. A person is overweight (350 pounds) and desires to lose 10% of his body weight over 6 months. Calculate the amount of total desired weight loss and amount of desired weight loss per month.

6. In question #5, what is the total kcalorie intake restriction required to reach the weight-loss goal? If the weight loss time period is 27 weeks, what are the weekly and daily kcalorie restrictions to achieve this goal?

7. A person has a BMI of 15.5 and desires to gain weight. Do you support the person's desire to gain weight based on the categorization of the BMI? If the person's EER is 2100, how many kcalories should be consumed per day to support weight gain of 1 pound per week?

8. A person has a BMI of 27 and needs to lose weight. If the person's EER is 2300 kcalories, how many kcalories per day should this person consume to promote weight loss? If the person had a BMI of 36, what would be the recommended daily energy intake for weight loss?

⑥ Chapter 9 Answer Key ⑥

Summing Up

1. number
2. fat
3. losses
4. set-point
5. interact
6. Environmental
7. inactivity
8. predisposition
9. factors
10. overweight
11. genetic
12. disease
13. overweight
14. overweight
15. supplements
16. obese
17. activity
18. aggressive
19. risks
20. combination
21. expended
22. modification
23. restructuring
24. time
25. registered dietitian
26. prevalent
27. increase
28. energy-dense

Chapter Study Questions

1. The prevalence of overweight and obesity has increased over the years and continues to be high. In the past 30 years, obesity increased in every state, in both genders, and across all ages, races, and educational levels. Approximately 68% of the adults in the U.S. are considered overweight or obese. The prevalence of overweight among children in the U.S. has also risen at a alarming rate as 34% of children are either overweight or obese. Obesity is widespread and is considered an epidemic.

2. When energy intake exceeds needs, fat cells within adipose tissues increase in size as triglycerides are added to them. Fat cells may increase in number as well, especially as existing cells are enlarged. Prevention of excess weight gain depends on maintaining a reasonable number of fat cells; when an obese person loses weight, the fat cells shrink, but their number does not decrease. Having these extra fat cells makes weight regain more rapid. According to set-point theory, the body attempts to return to the original weight, or its set point, after weight loss.

3. Genetics and epigenetics play a truly causative role in only a few cases of obesity. Genetics can predispose a person toward obesity or overweight. The hormone leptin (coded for by the *ob* gene) is involved in appetite and energy expenditure, and the hormone ghrelin triggers the desire to eat. Uncoupling proteins influence basal metabolic rate by uncoupling fat oxidation from ATP production within brown fat cells; the energy from oxidation is released as heat and thus is expended instead of being stored.

4. Environmental factors include everything outside the body that promote overeating and physical inactivity. An obesogenic environment includes all of the circumstances that are encountered daily that push people toward fatness. Overeating is encouraged by readily available, inexpensive, high-kcalorie foods and beverages that taste good and are served in large portions. Physical inactivity is facilitated by sedentary occupations, labor-saving devices, and the popularity of sedentary entertainments such as television and computer games.

5. Health professionals use a combination of weight status indicators—BMI and waist circumference—and disease risk profile to determine the desirability of weight loss for an individual. Weight loss is recommended for persons who are overweight or obese and who have 2 or more chronic disease risk factors (such as hypertension, smoking, etc.) and/or are suffering from a life-threatening condition such as diabetes. Weight loss may not be recommended when a person is overweight by standards but otherwise in good health. If the person's primary motivation for weight loss is vanity and not health promotion, and he/she opts for counterproductive strategies that are likely to result in regain, weight loss is not advisable.

6. Obese people face discrimination on the job, at school, and in social situations, where they are negatively stereotyped as lazy or lacking self-discipline; they often have psychological problems, including embarrassment in response to the prejudice of others and feelings of rejection, shame, and depression.

7. Fad diets are hazardous to health and can cause headaches, nausea, dizziness, and even death; weight-loss products are largely unregulated and may contain undeclared pharmaceutical ingredients that can cause seizures and heart attacks; other gimmicks that don't work include hot baths and saunas that may cause dehydration.

8. The drug orlistat is used to inhibit pancreatic lipase activity in the GI tract. This blocks digestion and absorption of dietary fat. Some side effects include cramping diarrhea, gas, frequent bowel movements, reduced absorption

of fat-soluble vitamins, and, in rare cases, liver injury. Phentermine, diethylpriopion, and phendimetrazine enhance the release of the neurotransmitter norepinephrine, which suppresses appetite. Side effects include increased blood pressure and heart rate, insomnia, nervousness, dizziness, and headache. When used as a part of a long-term, comprehensive weight-loss program, drugs can help with modest weight loss. Surgery is another aggressive option for weight loss. The gastric bypass procedure suppresses hunger by reducing production of GI hormones. In this procedure, the surgeon constructs a small stomach pouch that bypasses most of the stomach, the entire duodenum, and some of the jejunum. In both gastric bypass and gastric banding, the amount of food that can be comfortably eaten is limited. In gastric banding, the surgeon uses a gastric band to reduce the opening from the esophagus to the stomach. Liposuction removes body fat but has little effect on weight loss. These treatments may offer benefits but also incur some risks.

9. Eating plans for weight loss should be based on realistic energy intake and nutritional adequacy. Small portions of low-energy-density, high-fiber foods should be chosen and consumed at a leisurely pace with plenty of water. Total fat intake should be moderate, with mono- and polyunsaturated fats emphasized and saturated fats limited. Carbohydrate-rich foods should be chosen so as to incorporate fiber and restrict sugary foods high in empty kcalories. In addition, dietary strategies should be combined with non-dietary ones: physical activity, making small behavior modification changes, and support groups.

10. Physical activity burns kcalories, improves body composition, increases BMR, helps control appetite, and provides psychological benefits.

11. Behavioral strategies involve identifying the behaviors that have resulted in weight gain and replacing them with behaviors that increase energy expenditure and decrease energy intake. The individual should begin with small time-specific goals (e.g., adding 30 minutes of moderate activity to the daily routine) and practice new behaviors until they become habits. Successful changes are supported by the cognitive skills of problem solving (being able to identify problems and potential solutions) and cognitive restructuring (thinking positive, encouraging thoughts instead of self-defeating ones). It is also helpful to identify any particular stressors that trigger overeating and plan how to respond to them in a more healthful way.

12. People who are underweight (based on BMI) but in good health can safely remain at their current weight; those who are overly thin because of malnourishment or illness may benefit from weight gain. Causes of underweight include genetic tendencies, hunger and appetite problems, satiety irregularities, psychological traits, and metabolic factors. Food aversions and anorexia nervosa can also cause severe malnutrition.

13. Eat energy-dense foods to provide an excess of at least 500 kcal per day, consume regular meals daily, take large portions, eat extra snacks between meals, drink plenty of caloric beverages such as juice and milk, and perform strength-training exercises to build muscle.

Key Terms Practice

1. cellulite	5. underweight	9. d	13. f
2. fad diets	6. ghrelin	10. g	14. c
3. serotonin	7. epidemic	11. e	15. i
4. leptin	8. h	12. b	16. a

Sample Test Questions

1. b (p. 261)	9. a (p. 264)	17. a (pp. 268-269)	25. c (p. 279)
2. c (pp. 262, 263)	10. d (p. 264)	18. a (p. 273)	26. b (pp. 278-280)
3. d (p. 262)	11. d (pp. 268-269)	19. b (pp. 274-278)	27. a (p. 282)
4. a (p. 262)	12. e (p. 269)	20. a (p. 274)	28. d (p. 281)
5. b (pp. 262-263)	13. c (p. 271)	21. c (p. 276)	29. d (p. 286)
6. d (p. 262)	14. c (p. 266)	22. a (p. 277)	30. b (p. 284)
7. c (p. 265)	15. b (p. 271)	23. d (p. 276)	
8. d (p. 263)	16. a (pp. 271-272)	24. a (pp. 278-279)	

Short Answer Questions

1. underweight: <18.5; healthy weight: 18.5–24.9; overweight: 25.0–29.9; obese: ≥30

2. number, size

3. leptin, ghrelin

4. overeating, physical inactivity

5. body mass index, waist circumference, disease risk profile

6. the extent of overweight, age, health, genetic makeup

7. drugs (e.g., orlistate, phentermine), surgery (e.g., gastric bypass, gastric banding)

8. do not grocery shop when hungry; eat slowly (pause during meals, chew thoroughly, put down utensils between bites); exercise when watching television

9. short-term increase in energy expenditure; long-term increase in BMR (from an increase in lean tissue); improved body composition; appetite control; stress reduction and control of stress eating; physical, and therefore psychological, well-being; improved self-esteem

10. emphasize energy-dense foods (energy in should exceed energy out by at least 500 kcalories/day); exercise to build muscles; eat at least three meals a day; eat large portions of foods and expect to feel full; eat snacks between meals; drink plenty of juice and milk

Problem Solving

1. 35 kcal divided by 75 g = 0.47 kcal/g

2. 100 kcal divided by 60 g = 1.67 kcal/g

3. l lb. fat = 3500 kcal divided by 7 days/week = 500 kcal/day deficit
   4000 − 500 kcalories = 3500 kcalories/day
   210 − 175 pounds = 35 lb. = 35 weeks

4. 2 g × 7 kcal/g = 14 kcalories from alcohol
   60 g × 4 kcal/g = 240 kcalories from carbohydrate
   20 g × 4 kcal/g = 80 kcalories from protein
   40 g × 9 kcal/g = 360 kcalories from fat
   14 + 240 + 80 + 360 = 694 total kcalories

   This beverage is energy dense, is very high in fat, and likely provides many empty calories from fat, sugar, and alcohol without much satiety value. It would be appropriate on a weight-loss diet only as an occasional treat, and in a smaller portion than this.

5. 350 × 0.10 = desires to lose 35 pounds over 6 months. 35 divided by 6 months = 5.833 lb. per month.

6. 35 pounds × 3500 kcal/lb. = total restriction of 122,500 kcalories
   122,500 divided by 27 weeks = 4537 fewer kcal per week
   4537 divided by 7 = 648 fewer kcal per day

7. The BMI of 15.5 is less than 18.5 so the person is classified as underweight. Weight gain in this case may be appropriate for good health. 2100 + (500-1000) = 2600 to 3100 kcalories per day to support weight gain of 1 pound per week.

8. A person with a BMI of 27 should consume 300 to 500 kcalories per day less than his or her usual intake. 2300 kcal − 300-500 kcal = 1800-2000 kcal/day. A person with a BMI of 36 should decrease intake by 500 to 1000 kcal per day: 2300 kcal − 500-1000 kcal = 1300-1800 kcal/day.

⑥ Chapter 10 ~ The Water-Soluble Vitamins: ⑥ B Vitamins and Vitamin C

Chapter Outline

I. The Vitamins—An Overview
    A. Bioavailability
    B. Precursors
    C. Organic Nature
    D. Solubility
    E. Toxicity

II. The B Vitamins
    A. Thiamin
      1. Thiamin Recommendations
      2. Thiamin Deficiency and Toxicity
      3. Thiamin Food Sources
    B. Riboflavin
      1. Riboflavin Recommendations
      2. Riboflavin Deficiency and Toxicity
      3. Riboflavin Food Sources
    C. Niacin
      1. Niacin Recommendations
      2. Niacin Deficiency
      3. Niacin Toxicity
      4. Niacin Food Sources
    D. Biotin
      1. Biotin Recommendations
      2. Biotin Deficiency and Toxicity
      3. Biotin Food Sources
    E. Pantothenic Acid
      1. Pantothenic Acid Recommendations
      2. Pantothenic Acid Deficiency and Toxicity
      3. Pantothenic Acid Food Sources
    F. Vitamin B_6
      1. Vitamin B_6 Recommendations
      2. Vitamin B_6 Deficiency
      3. Vitamin B_6 Toxicity
      4. Vitamin B_6 Food Sources
    G. Folate
      1. Folate Recommendations
      2. Folate and Neural Tube Defects
      3. Folate and Heart Disease
      4. Folate and Cancer
      5. Folate Deficiency
      6. Folate Toxicity
      7. Folate Food Sources
    H. Vitamin B_{12}
      1. Vitamin B_{12} Recommendations
      2. Vitamin B_{12} Deficiency and Toxicity
      3. Vitamin B_{12} Food Sources

    I. Choline
      1. Choline Recommendations
      2. Choline Deficiency and Toxicity
      3. Choline Food Sources
    J. Nonvitamins
    K. Interactions among the B Vitamins
      1. B Vitamin Roles
      2. B Vitamin Deficiencies
      3. B Vitamin Toxicities
      4. B Vitamin Food Sources

III. Vitamin C
    A. Vitamin C Roles
      1. As an Antioxidant
      2. As a Cofactor in Collagen Formation
      3. As a Cofactor in Other Reactions
      4. In Stress
      5. In the Prevention and Treatment of the Common Cold
      6. In Disease Prevention
    B. Vitamin C Recommendations
    C. Vitamin C Deficiency
    D. Vitamin C Toxicity
    E. Vitamin C Food Sources

IV. Vitamin and Mineral Supplements
    A. Arguments for Supplements
      1. Correct Overt Deficiencies
      2. Support Increased Nutrient Needs
      3. Improve Nutrition Status
      4. Improve the Body's Defenses
      5. Reduce Disease Risks
      6. Who Needs Supplements?
    B. Arguments against Supplements
      1. Who Should Not Take Supplements?
      2. Toxicity
      3. Life-Threatening Misinformation
      4. Unknown Needs
      5. False Sense of Security
      6. Other Invalid Reasons
      7. Bioavailability and Antagonistic Actions
    C. Selection of Supplements
      1. Form
      2. Contents
      3. Misleading Claims
      4. Cost
    D. Regulation of Supplements

Summing Up

The 1._____ are essential nutrients needed in tiny amounts in the diet both to prevent 2._____ diseases and to support 3._____ health. The 4._____-_____ vitamins are the B vitamins and vitamin C; the 5._____-_____ vitamins are vitamins A, D, E, and 6.___.

The B vitamins serve as 7._____ that facilitate the work of every 8._____. They are active in carbohydrate, fat, and protein 9._____ and in the making of 10._____ and thus new cells. Historically famous B vitamin–deficiency diseases are 11._____ (thiamin), 12._____ (niacin), and 13._____ anemia (vitamin B$_{12}$). Pellagra can be prevented by adequate 14._____ because the amino acid tryptophan can be converted to 15._____ in the body. A high intake of folate can 16._____ the blood symptoms of a vitamin B$_{12}$ deficiency, but it will not prevent the associated 17._____ damage. Vitamin B$_6$ participates in 18._____ acid metabolism and can be 19._____ in excess. Biotin and pantothenic acid serve important roles in 20._____ metabolism and are common in a variety of foods. Many 21._____ that people claim as B vitamins are not. Fortunately, a variety of foods from each of the food groups provides an 22._____ supply of all of the B vitamins.

Vitamin C acts primarily as an 23._____ and a cofactor. Recommendations are set well 24._____ the amount needed to prevent the deficiency disease 25._____. A variety of fruits and vegetables—most notably 26._____ fruits—provide generous amounts of vitamin C.

Chapter Study Questions

1. How do the vitamins differ from the energy nutrients?

2. Describe some general differences between fat-soluble and water-soluble vitamins.

3. Which B vitamins are involved in energy metabolism? Protein metabolism? Cell division?

124

4. For thiamin, riboflavin, niacin, biotin, pantothenic acid, vitamin B_6, folate, and vitamin B_{12}, state:
   - Its chief function in the body.
   - Its characteristic deficiency symptoms.
   - Its significant food sources.

5. What is the relationship between tryptophan and niacin?

6. Describe the relationship between folate and vitamin B_{12}.

4. For vitamin C state:
   - Its chief function in the body.
   - Its characteristic deficiency symptoms.
   - Its significant food sources.

8. What risks are associated with high doses of niacin? Vitamin B_6? Vitamin C?

Key Terms Practice

To complete the crossword puzzle, identify the key term that best matches each definition.

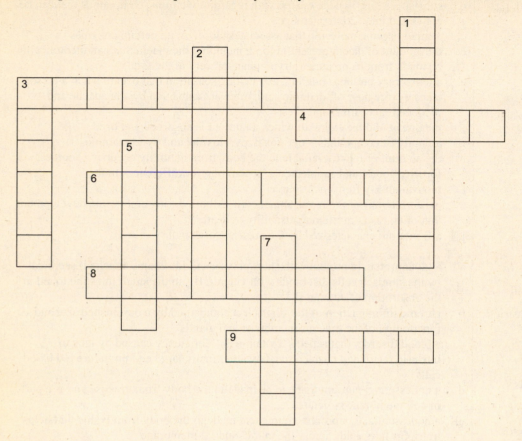

Across:
3. The thiamin-deficiency disease.
4. A B vitamin; also known as folic acid, folacin, or pteroylglutamic acid.
6. A competing factor that counteracts the action of another factor.
8. Organic, essential nutrients required in tiny amounts to perform specific functions that promote growth, reproduction, or the maintenance of health and life.
9. The vitamin C–deficiency disease.

Down:
1. A small, inorganic or organic substance that facilitates the action of an enzyme.
2. The niacin-deficiency disease.
3. A B vitamin that functions as a coenzyme in metabolism.
5. A condition in which too few red blood cells are present, or the red blood cells are immature (and therefore large) or too small or contain too little hemoglobin to carry the normal amount of oxygen to the tissues.
7. A B vitamin that can be made in the body from its precursor, tryptophan, an essential amino acid.

Match the key terms with their definitions.

10. _____ bioavailability	a.	a B vitamin whose principal active form is part of coenzyme A
11. _____ coenzyme	b.	substances that precede others; with regard to vitamins, compounds that can be converted into active vitamins
12. _____ dietary folate equivalents	c.	a small organic molecule that associates closely with certain enzymes
	d.	the amount of niacin present in food, including the niacin that can theoretically be made from its precursor, tryptophan, present in the food
13. _____ neural tube defects	e.	a temporary burning, tingling, and itching sensation that occurs when a person takes a large dose of nicotinic acid; often accompanied by a headache and reddened face, arms, and chest
14. _____ niacin equivalents		
15. _____ niacin flush	f.	the rate at and the extent to which a nutrient is absorbed and used
16. _____ pantothenic acid	g.	a family of compounds—pyridoxal, pyridoxine, and pyridoxamine
17. _____ precursors	h.	the amount of folate available to the body from naturally occurring sources, fortified foods, and supplements, accounting for differences in the bioavailability from each source
18. _____ vitamin B_6	i.	malformations of the brain, spinal cord, or both during embryonic development that often result in lifelong disability or death
19. _____ vitamin B_{12}	j.	a B vitamin characterized by the presence of cobalt

20. _____ antioxidant	a.	a glycoprotein (a protein with short polysaccharide chains attached) secreted by the stomach cells that binds with vitamin B_{12} in the small intestine to aid in the absorption of vitamin B_{12}
21. _____ ascorbic acid		
22. _____ atrophic gastritis	b.	chronic inflammation of the stomach accompanied by a diminished size and functioning of the mucous membrane and glands
23. _____ carnitine	c.	a blood disorder that reflects a vitamin B_{12} deficiency caused by lack of intrinsic factor and characterized by abnormally large and immature red blood cells
24. _____ collagen		
25. _____ free radicals	d.	a nonessential nutrient that can be made in the body from glucose and is a part of cell membrane structures
26. _____ inositol		
27. _____ intrinsic factor	e.	a nonessential, nonprotein amino acid made in the body from lysine that helps transport fatty acids across the mitochondrial membrane
28. _____ oxidative stress	f.	one of the two active forms of vitamin C
29. _____ pernicious anemia	g.	a substance in foods that significantly decreases the adverse effects of free radicals on normal physiological functions in the human body
	h.	unstable molecules with one or more unpaired electrons
	i.	a condition in which the production of oxidants and free radicals exceeds the body's ability to handle them and prevent damage
	j.	the structural protein from which connective tissues such as scars, tendons, ligaments, and the foundations of bones and teeth are made

Sample Test Questions

Select the best answer for each question.

1. Vitamins are:
   a. organic.
   b. inorganic.
   c. essential nutrients required in small amounts.
   d. a and c
   e. b and c

2. How do vitamins differ from carbohydrates, protein, and fat?
   a. Function
   b. Structure
   c. Amounts required
   d. a and c only
   e. a, b, and c

3. How are vitamins similar to carbohydrates, protein, and fat?
   a. They have similar functions.
   b. They are vital to life.
   c. They are organic.
   d. a and b
   e. b and c

4. A measure of the amount of vitamins absorbed and used by the body is called:
   a. bioavailability.
   b. dissolvability.
   c. solubility.
   d. utilization.

5. The body's ability to use vitamins is affected by:
   a. time of transit through the GI tract.
   b. previous nutrient intake.
   c. method of food preparation.
   d. a and b
   e. a, b and c

6. Some vitamins that are present in inactive forms are called:
   a. synthetics.
   b. precursors.
   c. organics.
   d. elements.

7. To minimize nutrient losses from fruits and vegetables:
   a. keep them on kitchen counters.
   b. cook them very thoroughly.
   c. store them in airtight containers.
   d. cook them in large amounts of water.

8. Which nutrients are hydrophilic?
   a. All vitamins
   b. B vitamins
   c. Fat-soluble vitamins
   d. Lipids

9. Water-soluble vitamins consumed in excess of need may be:
   a. malabsorbed.
   b. beneficial.
   c. harmful.
   d. a and b
   e. a and c

10. B vitamins:
    a. are water soluble.
    b. function as coenzymes.
    c. are stored in the adipose tissue.
    d. are absorbed into the lymph.
    e. a and b

11. A dietary deficiency of B vitamins can cause:
    a. negative nitrogen balance.
    b. impairment of energy metabolism.
    c. impaired iron utilization.
    d. reduced thyroid production.

12. A prolonged deficiency of thiamin produces the disease:
    a. rickets.
    b. pellagra.
    c. beriberi.
    d. scurvy.

13. Which of the following deficiencies is observed in most alcohol abusers?
    a. Thiamin
    b. Niacin
    c. Folate
    d. Vitamin B_6

14. Which of the following vitamins is most readily destroyed by ultraviolet light?
    a. Niacin
    b. Thiamin
    c. Riboflavin
    d. Ascorbic acid

15. The dietary need for _____ is influenced by the presence of the amino acid tryptophan in the diet.
    a. thiamin
    b. pantothenic acid
    c. niacin
    d. biotin
    e. riboflavin

16. Two coenzyme forms of niacin are:
    a. FMN and FAD.
    b. NAD and FAD.
    c. NADP and TPP.
    d. FAD and TPP.
    e. NADP and NAD.

17. The disease called pellagra is related to a:
    a. dietary deficiency of riboflavin.
    b. low-protein diet high in corn products.
    c. diet high in polished rice.
    d. a and b
    e. a and c

18. Which of the following is highest in riboflavin content per serving?
    a. Butter
    b. Milk
    c. Bread
    d. Apple
    e. Egg

19. If your skin tingles, itches, and turns red after you take a vitamin pill you may have overdosed on:
    a. niacin.
    b. thiamin.
    c. riboflavin.
    d. folate.

20. Pantothenic acid is a part of the structure of:
    a. pyruvate.
    b. NADP.
    c. cobalamin.
    d. pyridoxal phosphate.
    e. coenzyme A.

21. Which of the following statements is **true** about vitamin B_6?
    a. It is stored exclusively in fat tissue.
    b. It enhances athletic performance, especially endurance.
    c. It cures premenstrual syndrome.
    d. It may cause irreversible nerve damage in large doses.

22. Often a function of one vitamin depends on the presence of another. This interdependence is shown in which two vitamins?
    a. Vitamin B_{12} and folate
    b. Vitamin A and vitamin C
    c. Vitamin B_{12} and niacin
    d. Folate and vitamin C

23. Vitamin B_{12} is different from other B vitamins because:
    a. it may be synthesized from a certain amino acid.
    b. it requires a carrier to be transported from the intestinal tract to the bloodstream.
    c. deficiencies of vitamin B_{12} never occur in human beings.
    d. it is found only in plant foods.

24. _____ will be lacking in the diet of strict vegetarians (vegans) who do not use fortified foods or supplements.
    a. Vitamin B_{12}
    b. Thiamin
    c. Riboflavin
    d. Niacin
    e. Biotin

25. Folate has proven critical in reducing the risks of:
    a. learning disabilities.
    b. alcoholism.
    c. neural tube defects.
    d. ADD.

26. The best food source of folate among the following is:
    a. spinach.
    b. milk.
    c. coffee.
    d. ice cream.

27. The vitamin C deficiency disease is:
    a. ascorbic acidosis.
    b. scurvy.
    c. pellagra.
    d. beriberi.

28. Most of the symptoms of a vitamin C deficiency are caused by:
    a. anemia.
    b. failure to maintain integrity of blood vessels.
    c. inactivity of intestinal bacteria.
    d. decreased utilization of protein.

29. The amount of vitamin C needed to prevent overt deficiency symptoms is about:
    a. 10 milligrams a day.
    b. 35 milligrams a day.
    c. 60 milligrams a day.
    d. 100 milligrams a day.

30. Which of the following is lowest in vitamin C?
    a. Strawberries
    b. Potatoes
    c. Milk
    d. Broccoli
    e. Orange juice

Short Answer Questions

1. General characteristics of water-soluble vitamins are:

    a.   d.

    b.   e.

    c.   f.

2. The names of the water-soluble vitamins are:

    a.   f.

    b.   g.

    c.   h.

    d.   i.

    e.

3. Distinguish between these types of deficiencies:

    a. primary:

    b. secondary:

4. B vitamins are active in metabolism of these nutrients:

    a.   c.

    b.

5. Historically famous B-vitamin deficiency diseases are:

    a.   c.

    b.

6. Chief roles of vitamin B$_6$ include:

    a.

    b.

    c.

7. Vitamin C act primarily as:

    a.   b.

8. Excess amounts of vitamin C may obscure results of urine tests and cause:

    a.   b.

Problem Solving

1. A person whose RDA for protein is 45 grams consumes 75 grams of protein in a day. How many niacin equivalents does this represent?

2. A 35-year-old man consumed the following folate-containing foods for lunch: a sandwich made with 2 slices of fortified bread (14 µg natural, 48 µg synthetic) and 4 tablespoons peanut butter (47 µg); ½ cup carrot sticks (12 µg); an orange (48 µg); and 2 graham crackers (5 µg natural, 8 µg synthetic). What percentage of his RDA for folate did his lunch provide?

3. What percentage of the RDA for vitamin C does a female nonsmoker receive from ½ cup of broccoli (40.6 mg vitamin C)?

❦ Chapter 10 Answer Key ❦

Summing Up

1. vitamins	8. cell	15. niacin	22. adequate
2. deficiency	9. metabolism	16. mask	23. antioxidant
3. optimal	10. DNA	17. nerve	24. above
4. water-soluble	11. beriberi	18. amino	25. scurvy
5. fat-soluble	12. pellagra	19. harmful	26. citrus
6. K	13. pernicious	20. energy	
7. coenzymes	14. protein	21. substances	

Chapter Study Questions

1. They differ in structure (they are individual units and not linked together), function (they don't yield energy), and the units of measurement used to express food contents (they occur in much smaller quantities in foods).

2. Typically, water-soluble vitamins are: absorbed directly into and circulate freely in the blood and other watery fluids; excreted in the urine; needed in frequent, small doses; and unlikely to reach toxic levels in the body. Fat-soluble vitamins are: absorbed into the lymph and carried in the blood by protein carriers, stored in body fat, needed in periodic doses, and more likely to be toxic when consumed in excess of needs.

3. B vitamins involved in energy metabolism: thiamin, riboflavin, niacin, biotin, and pantothenic acid. B vitamin involved in protein metabolism: vitamin B_6. B vitamins involved in cell division: folate and vitamin B_{12}.

4. See text for respective summary tables for each nutrient (pp. 303, 304, 308, 309, 311, 315, and 318).

5. Tryptophan can be converted to niacin in the body: 60 mg tryptophan = 1 mg niacin.

6. Vitamin B_{12} and folate's roles intertwine because each depends on the other for activation. Folate is part of a coenzyme that helps transfer 1-C compounds, an action necessary to convert vitamin B_{12} to one of its coenzyme forms. Vitamin B_{12} removes a methyl group to activate the folate coenzyme; when folate gives up its methyl group, the vitamin B_{12} enzyme is activated. Both folate and vitamin B_{12} are required for synthesis of DNA and RNA and the regeneration of the amino acid methionine from homocysteine.

7. See text for summary table for vitamin C (p. 327).

8. Niacin: painful flush, hives, and rash ("niacin flush"); nausea and vomiting; liver damage; and impaired glucose tolerance. Vitamin B_6: depression, fatigue, irritability, headaches, nerve damage (causing numbness, muscle weakness leading to an inability to walk and convulsions), and skin lesions. Vitamin C: nausea, abdominal cramps, diarrhea, headache, fatigue, insomnia, hot flashes, rashes, interference with medical tests, aggravation of gout symptoms, urinary tract problems, kidney stones.

Key Terms Practice

1. cofactor	8. vitamins	16. a	24. j
2. pellagra	9. scurvy	17. b	25. h
3. A: beriberi;	10. f	18. g	26. d
D: biotin	11. c	19. j	27. a
4. folate	12. h	20. g	28. i
5. anemia	13. i	21. f	29. c
6. antagonist	14. d	22. b	
7. niacin	15. e	23. e	

Sample Test Questions

1. d (p. 297)	9. c (pp. 299-300)	16. e (p. 305)	24. a (p. 317)
2. e (p. 298)	10. e (pp. 298, 300)	17. b (pp. 305-306)	25. c (p. 313)
3. e (p. 297)	11. b (pp. 300, 319-320)	18. b (pp. 304, 305)	26. a (p. 315)
4. a (p. 298)		19. a (p. 306)	27. b (p. 322)
5. e (p. 298)	12. c (p. 301)	20. e (p. 308)	28. b (p. 325)
6. b (p. 298)	13. a (p. 301)	21. d (p. 310)	29. a (p. 324)
7. c (p. 299)	14. c (p. 304)	22. a (pp. 310, 315)	30. c (p. 326)
8. b (p. 298)	15. c (p. 305)	23. b (pp. 315-316)	

Short Answer Questions

1. absorbed directly into the blood; transported freely in the body; circulate freely in water-filled compartments; excreted in urine; less likely to be toxic (compared to fat-soluble vitamins); needed in frequent doses

2. thiamin, riboflavin, niacin, biotin, pantothenic acid, vitamin B_6, folate, vitamin B_{12}, vitamin C

3. a. results from inadequate intake; b. results from causes other than level of intake, such as impaired absorption or an unusual metabolic need

4. carbohydrate, protein, fat

5. beriberi, pellagra, pernicious anemia

6. amino acid and fatty acid metabolism; conversion of tryptophan to niacin and serotonin; red blood cell production (heme synthesis)

7. an antioxidant, a cofactor (in the synthesis of collagen and other compounds)

8. false positives, false negatives

Problem Solving

1. 75 g - 45 g = 30 g excess protein
   30 g divided by 100 = 0.3 g tryptophan
   0.3 g × 1000 mg/g = 300 mg tryptophan
   300 mg divided by 60 = 5 mg niacin equivalents

2. DFE = 14 µg + 47 µg + 12 µg + 48 µg + 5 µg + 1.7 × (48 µg + 8 µg)
   DFE = 126 µg + 1.7 × 56 µg = 126 µg + 95.2 µg = 221 µg DFE
   221 µg DFE divided by 400 µg DFE (RDA for adults) = 55%

3. RDA for nonsmoking female adults = 75 mg
   40.6 mg divided by 75 mg = 54%

❧ Chapter 11 – The Fat-Soluble Vitamins: ❧ A, D, E, and K

Chapter Outline

I. Vitamin A and Beta-Carotene
   A. Roles in the Body
      1. Vitamin A in Vision
      2. Vitamin A in Protein Synthesis and Cell Differentiation
      3. Vitamin A in Reproduction and Growth
      4. Beta-Carotene as an Antioxidant
   B. Vitamin A Deficiency
      1. Infectious Diseases
      2. Night Blindness
      3. Blindness (Xerophthalmia)
      4. Keratinization
   C. Vitamin A Toxicity
      1. Bone Defects
      2. Birth Defects
      3. Not for Acne
   D. Vitamin A Recommendations
   E. Vitamin A in Foods
      1. The Colors of Vitamin A Foods
      2. Vitamin A-Rich Liver
II. Vitamin D
   A. Roles in the Body
      1. Vitamin D in Bone Growth
      2. Vitamin D in Other Roles
   B. Vitamin D Deficiency
      1. Rickets
      2. Osteomalacia
      3. Osteoporosis
      4. The Elderly
   C. Vitamin D Toxicity
   D. Vitamin D Recommendations and Sources
      1. Vitamin D in Foods
      2. Vitamin D from the Sun
      3. Vitamin D from Supplements
III. Vitamin E
   A. Vitamin E as an Antioxidant
   B. Vitamin E Deficiency
   C. Vitamin E Toxicity
   D. Vitamin E Recommendations
   E. Vitamin E in Foods
IV. Vitamin K
   A. Roles in the Body
   B. Vitamin K Deficiency
   C. Vitamin K Toxicity
   D. Vitamin K Recommendations and Sources
V. Antioxidant Nutrients in Disease Prevention
   A. Free Radicals and Disease
   B. Defending against Free Radicals
   C. Defending against Cancer
   D. Defending against Heart Disease
   E. Foods, Supplements, or Both?

Summing Up

Vitamin A is found in the body in three forms: retinol, 1._____, and retinoic acid. Together, they are essential to 2._____, healthy epithelial tissues, and 3._____. Vitamin A deficiency is a major health problem worldwide, leading to 4._____, blindness, and 5._____. Toxicity can also cause problems and is most often associated with 6._____ abuse. Animal-derived foods such as liver and whole or fortified milk provide 7._____, whereas brightly colored plant-derived foods such as spinach, carrots, and pumpkins provide 8._____-_____ and other carotenoids. In addition to serving as a 9._____ for vitamin A, beta-carotene acts as an 10._____ in the body.

Vitamin D can be synthesized in the body with the help of 11._____ or obtained from some foods, most notably 12._____ milk. Vitamin D sends signals to three primary target sites: the GI tract to absorb more 13._____ and phosphorus, the 14._____ to release more, and the kidneys to 15._____ more. These actions maintain blood 16._____ concentrations and support bone formation. A deficiency causes 17._____ in childhood and 18._____ in later life.

Vitamin E acts as an antioxidant, defending 19._____ and other components of the cells against 20._____ damage. Deficiencies are rare, but they do occur in 21._____ infants, the primary symptom being erythrocyte 22._____. Vitamin E is found predominantly in 23._____ oils and appears to be one of the 24._____ toxic of the fat-soluble vitamins.

Vitamin K helps with blood 25._____, and its deficiency causes hemorrhagic disease (uncontrolled 26._____). Bacteria in the GI tract can make the vitamin; people typically receive about half of their requirements from 27._____ synthesis and half from foods such as 28._____ vegetables and vegetable oils. Because people depend on bacterial 29._____ for vitamin K, deficiency is most likely in newborn infants and in people taking 30._____.

Chapter Study Questions

1. List the fat-soluble vitamins. What characteristics do they have in common? How do they differ from the water-soluble vitamins?

2. Summarize the roles of vitamin A and the symptoms of its deficiency.

3. What is meant by *vitamin precursors*? Name the precursors of vitamin A, and tell in what classes of foods they are located. Give examples of foods with high vitamin A activity.

4. Describe potential outcomes of vitamin A toxicity.

5. How is vitamin D unique among the vitamins? What is its chief function? What are the richest sources of this vitamin?

6. What are toxic effects of vitamin D? What causes vitamin D toxicity?

7. Describe vitamin E's role as an antioxidant. What are the chief symptoms of vitamin E deficiency?

8. Discuss vitamin E's potential for toxicity. What food sources provide significant amounts of vitamin E?

9. What are vitamin K's primary roles in the body? What conditions may lead to vitamin K deficiency?

10. What is known about vitamin K toxicity? What sources provide significant amounts of vitamin K?

Key Terms Practice

To complete the crossword puzzle, identify the key term that best matches each definition.

Across:

3. A molecule capable of absorbing certain wavelengths of light so that it reflects only those that we perceive as a certain color.
4. A water-insoluble protein normally present in hair and nails.
7. The transparent membrane covering the outside of the eye.
9. A calcium-binding protein in bones, essential for normal mineralization.
10. A chronic inflammation of the skin's follicles and oil-producing glands, which leads to an accumulation of oils inside the ducts that surround hairs; usually associated with the maturation of young adults.

Down:

1. Free of microorganisms, such as bacteria.
2. The vitamin D-deficiency disease in children characterized by inadequate mineralization of bone (manifested in bowed legs or knock-knees, outward-bowed chest, and knobs on ribs).
5. Chemically related compounds with biological activity similar to that of retinol; metabolites of retinol.
6. Abnormal drying of the skin and mucous membranes; a sign of vitamin A deficiency.
8. The innermost membrane of the eye, composed of several layers including one that contains the rods and cones.

Match the key terms with their definitions.

11. _____ alpha-tocopherol

12. _____ beta-carotene

13. _____ cell differentiation

14. _____ epithelial cells

15. _____ epithelial tissue

16. _____ erythrocyte hemolysis

17. _____ hemolytic anemia

18. _____ mucous membranes

19. _____ retinol-binding protein

20. _____ vitamin A

a. the layer of the body that serves as a selective barrier between the body's interior and the environment
b. one of the carotenoids; an orange pigment and vitamin A precursor found in plants
c. the specific protein responsible for transporting retinol
d. the process by which immature cells develop specific functions different from those of the original that are characteristic of their mature cell type
e. cells on the surface of the skin and mucous membranes
f. all naturally occurring compounds with the biological activity of retinol, the alcohol form of vitamin A
g. the membranes, composed of mucus-secreting cells, that line the surfaces of body tissues
h. the active vitamin E compound
i. the breaking open of red blood cells; a symptom of vitamin E-deficiency disease in human beings
j. the condition of having too few red blood cells as a result of erythrocyte hemolysis

21. _____ cholecalciferol

22. _____ ergocalciferol

23. _____ keratinization

24. _____ keratomalacia

25. _____ night blindness

26. _____ osteomalacia

27. _____ preformed vitamin A

28. _____ retinol activity equivalents

29. _____ tocopherol

30. _____ xerophthalmia

a. a measure of vitamin A activity; the amount of retinol that the body will derive from a food containing preformed retinol or its precursor beta-carotene
b. accumulation of keratin in a tissue; a sign of vitamin A deficiency
c. slow recovery of vision after flashes of bright light at night or an inability to see in dim light; an early symptom of vitamin A deficiency
d. progressive blindness caused by inadequate tear production due to severe vitamin A deficiency
e. softening of the cornea that leads to irreversible blindness; seen in severe vitamin A deficiency
f. dietary vitamin A in its active form
g. vitamin D_2 derived from plants in the diet and made from the yeast and plant sterol ergosterol
h. vitamin D_3 derived from animals in the diet or made in the skin from 7-dehydrocholesterol, a precursor of cholesterol, with the help of sunlight
i. a bone disease characterized by softening of the bones; symptoms include bending of the spine and bowing of the legs
j. a general term for several chemically related compounds, one of which has vitamin E activity

Sample Test Questions

Select the best answer for each question.

1. A characteristic of the fat-soluble vitamins is that excesses are stored:
    a. in the liver and fatty tissues.
    b. in the blood.
    c. in epithelial cells.
    d. in mucous membranes.

2. _____ is the form of vitamin A that functions as an intermediate between other forms in the body.
    a. Retinol
    b. Retinal
    c. Retinoic acid
    d. Retinyl ester

3. Night vision is maintained by:
    a. vitamin A, which combines with opsin in the dark to regenerate rhodopsin.
    b. vitamin D, which combines with opsin in the dark to regenerate rhodopsin.
    c. vitamin A, which combines with rhodopsin in the dark to regenerate *trans*-retinal and opsin.
    d. vitamin E, which protects the polyunsaturated fatty acids in the membranes of the rod cells.

4. Which of the following surfaces is (are) **not** lined with epithelial cells?
    a. Bladder and urethra
    b. Mouth, stomach, and intestines
    c. Eyelids
    d. Lungs
    e. Bones

5. Which vitamin is needed for bones to grow in length?
    a. Vitamin A
    b. Vitamin B_1
    c. Vitamin C
    d. Vitamin D

6. The active forms of vitamin A in the body are:
    a. retinol, retinal, and retinoic acid.
    b. retinol, retinyl esters, and opsin.
    c. retinol, retinal, and carotenoids.
    d. all of the above

7. Retinol-binding protein:
    a. converts retinol to retinal.
    b. converts retinyl esters to retinol.
    c. cleaves beta-carotene.
    d. carries vitamin A in the blood.

8. Cell differentiation refers to:
    a. the action of mucous membranes.
    b. the process by which immature cells develop specific functions.
    c. the ability of cells to serve as selective barriers.
    d. dismantling of a structure.

9. What is a vitamin A precursor found in plants?
    a. Chlorophyll
    b. Beta-carotene
    c. Lysosome
    d. None of the above

10. The selective barrier between the body's interior and the environment is:
    a. epithelial tissue.
    b. the retina.
    c. the mucous membranes.
    d. tocopherol.

11. An early sign of vitamin A deficiency is:
    a. rickets.
    b. hemolytic anemia.
    c. night blindness.
    d. total blindness.

12. Which of the following is a symptom of a vitamin A deficiency?
    a. Anemia
    b. Fissuring at the corners of the mouth
    c. Keratinization of the epithelial cells
    d. Erythematous areas closely resembling sunburn appearing on the skin

13. Vitamin A toxicity:
    a. can pose a teratogenic risk.
    b. is impossible.
    c. is helpful for clearing up acne.
    d. None of the above

14. Among fruits and vegetables, the best sources of vitamin A are those that are:
    a. green or yellow, such as lettuce and corn.
    b. dark green or deep orange, such as broccoli and sweet potatoes.
    c. green, such as lettuce, peas, and snap beans.
    d. brightly colored, such as tomatoes and lemons.

15. Ultraviolet rays from the sun allow what vitamin to be synthesized?
    a. Vitamin A
    b. Vitamin B$_{12}$
    c. Vitamin C
    d. Vitamin D

16. Which of the following statements is true about vitamin D?
    a. It must be provided in the diet.
    b. It is an inorganic compound.
    c. It can be made in the body.
    d. It is not needed in adulthood.

17. The most important physiological function of vitamin D is:
    a. synthesis of red blood cells.
    b. promotion of calcium and phosphorus utilization.
    c. increased resistance to disease.
    d. prevention of night blindness.

18. The vitamin D-deficiency disease of children is:
    a. xerophthalmia.
    b. night blindness.
    c. follicular hyperkeratosis.
    d. rickets.

19. The major role of vitamin E in the body is to:
    a. aid in normal blood clotting.
    b. act as an antioxidant.
    c. aid in formation of normal epithelial tissue.
    d. aid in protein metabolism.

20. A symptom of vitamin E deficiency that has been demonstrated in human beings is:
    a. weak bones.
    b. muscle paralysis.
    c. reproductive failure.
    d. breakage of red blood cell membranes.

21. A condition of having too few red blood cells resulting from erythrocyte hemolysis is:
    a. muscular dystrophy.
    b. fibrocystic breast disease.
    c. hemorrhagic disease.
    d. hemolytic anemia.

22. A disease characterized by an inability of the blood to synthesize clotting factors is:
    a. hemolytic anemia.
    b. osteomalacia.
    c. hemophilia.
    d. intermittent claudication.

23. Vitamin E may reduce the risk of heart disease by protecting _____ against oxidation.
    a. low-density lipoproteins
    b. niacin
    c. brown fat cells
    d vitamin A

24. Vitamin E treatment:
    a. can cure hereditary muscular dystrophy in humans.
    b. if excessive, may interfere with blood clotting.
    c. is recommended for most people.
    d. is safe.

25. Vitamin E need varies with a person's intake of:
    a. polyunsaturated fatty acids.
    b. saturated fatty acids.
    c. cholesterol.
    d. other fat-soluble vitamins.

26. Vitamin K is necessary for:
    a. normal vision.
    b. normal blood clotting.
    c. normal muscle growth.
    d. normal cell differentiation.

27. If vitamin K is lacking, what condition may develop?
    a. Thrombosis
    b. Hemophilia
    c. Hemorrhagic disease
    d. All of the above

28. A vitamin K deficiency may occur as a result of:
    a. reduced fat absorption.
    b. antibiotic use.
    c. lack of sunlight.
    d. a and b
    e. a and c

29. Some of our vitamin K requirement is met by:
    a. synthesis of the vitamin by intestinal bacteria.
    b. synthesis of the vitamin from sunlight.
    c. synthesis of the vitamin from carotene.
    d. fortification of milk.

30. Toxicity of vitamin K:
    a. may cause death.
    b. is not common.
    c. may reduce the effectiveness of anticoagulant drugs.
    d. a and c
    e. b and c

Short Answer Questions

1. Characteristics of fat-soluble vitamins include:

    a.

    b.

    c.

    d.

2. The names of the fat-soluble vitamins are:

    a.

    b.

    c.

    d.

3. The three major roles of vitamin A are:

   a.

   b.

   c.

4. Four serious problems associated with vitamin A deficiencies are:

   a.   c.

   b.   d.

5. The two major negative consequences of vitamin A toxicity are:

   a.   b.

6. The major function of vitamin D is: _____

7. Three deficiency diseases of vitamin D are:

   a.   c.

   b.

8. The major role of vitamin E is: _____

9. The classic sign of vitamin E deficiency is: _____

10. The major role of vitamin K is: _____

11. Two circumstances in which a secondary deficiency of vitamin K may occur are:

    a.   b.

Problem Solving

1. If a carrot has 7,930 IU of beta-carotene, approximately how many μg RAE does it provide? If a supplement contains 20,000 IU of beta-carotene, approximately how many μg RAE does it provide?

2. If 3 oz. of liver provides 6,582 μg RAE, what percentage of the RDA for vitamin A does an adult female receive from 1 oz. of liver?

❧ Chapter 11 Answer Key ❧

Summing Up

1. retinal
2. vision
3. growth
4. infections
5. keratinization
6. supplement
7. retinoids
8. beta-carotene
9. precursor
10. antioxidant
11. sunlight
12. fortified
13. calcium
14. bones
15. retain
16. calcium
17. rickets
18. osteomalacia
19. lipids
20. oxidative
21. premature
22. hemolysis
23. vegetable
24. least
25. clotting
26. bleeding
27. bacterial
28. green
29. synthesis
30. antibiotics

Chapter Study Questions

1. Vitamins A, D, E, and K. Found in the fat and oily parts of foods; stored primarily in the liver and adipose tissue. Unlike water-soluble vitamins, fat-soluble ones require bile for digestion and are absorbed into the lymphatic system. Fat-soluble vitamins are stored longer and are less readily excreted; therefore, daily intake is less crucial and toxicity risk is greater than for water-soluble vitamins.

2. Vitamin A is important in vision; maintenance of the cornea, epithelial cells, mucous membranes, and skin; bone and tooth growth; reproduction; and immunity. Symptoms of deficiency include impaired immunity resulting in frequent respiratory, digestive, bladder, vaginal and other infections; night blindness, keratinization, and corneal degeneration leading to blindness (xerophthalmia); and plugging of hair follicles with keratin, forming white lumps (hyperkeratosis).

3. Compounds that can be converted into the active form of a vitamin. The vitamin A precursors—carotenoids (the most active being beta-carotene)—are available from plant foods; retinol compounds are available from animal foods. Examples of high-vitamin A activity foods are those with beta-carotene including spinach, winter squash, cantaloupe, carrots, sweet potatoes, and mangoes.

4. Excess vitamin A intake over the years may weaken the bones and contribute to fractures and osteoporosis. During pregnancy, excess vitamin A leads to abnormal cell death in the spinal cord, which increases the risk of birth defects.

5. With sunlight, vitamin D can be made from cholesterol (i.e., it is conditionally essential while the other vitamins are essential). Its chief function is to serve as a hormone to promote mineralization of bones and maintain blood mineral concentrations. Endogenous synthesis is a major source for healthy people with adequate sunlight exposure. The richest food sources are fortified milk, fortified margarine, eggs, liver, and fatty fish.

6. Vitamin D toxicity raises the concentration of blood calcium, which precipitates in the soft tissue, forming stones, especially in the kidneys where calcium is concentrated. Calcification may also harden the blood vessels and is especially dangerous in the major arteries of the brain, heart, and lungs, where it can cause death. The quantities of vitamin D found in foods and produced in the skin are well within normal recommendations; vitamin D supplements can contain toxic amounts.

7. Vitamin E protects other substances from oxidation by being oxidized itself; it protects the lipids and other vulnerable components of the cell and its membranes from destruction. It is especially effective in preventing the oxidation of the polyunsaturated fatty acids. Deficiency symptoms include red blood cell breakage (erythrocyte hemolysis) and anemia, as well as neuromuscular dysfunction involving the spinal cord and eye.

8. Toxicity of vitamin E appears to be rare and a broad range of intakes are considered safe. Extremely high doses of vitamin E may interfere with the blood clotting action of vitamin K and enhance the effects of drugs used to oppose blood clotting, causing hemorrhage. Vitamin E is widespread in foods. It occurs in vegetable oils and products made from them such as margarine and salad dressings. Wheat germ oil is especially rich in vitamin E. Other sources include spinach, turnip greens, collard greens, broccoli, wheat germ, whole grains, liver, egg yolks, nuts, seeds, and fatty meats.

9. Synthesis of blood-clotting proteins and bone proteins. Conditions that can lead to vitamin K deficiency include fat malabsorption and taking of antibiotics or anticoagulants while consuming a diet low in vitamin K. Newborn infants who do not receive a dose of vitamin K at birth are at risk for the first few weeks of life.

10. Vitamin K toxicity is not common and no adverse effects have been reported with high intakes of vitamin K. High doses of vitamin K can reduce the effectiveness of anticoagulant drugs use to prevent blood clotting. Vitamin K is made in the GI tract by resident bacteria. This provides about half of a person's needs. Vitamin K-rich foods such as green vegetables and vegetable oils supply the other half.

Key Terms Practice

1. sterile	9. osteocalcin	17. j	25. c
2. rickets	10. acne	18. g	26. i
3. pigment	11. h	19. c	27. f
4. keratin	12. b	20. f	28. a
5. retinoids	13. d	21. h	29. j
7. cornea	14. e	22. g	30. d
6. xerosis	15. a	23. b	
8. retina	16. i	24. e	

Sample Test Questions

1. a (p. 339)	9. b (p. 340)	17. b (pp. 347-348)	25. a (p. 354)
2. b (p. 341)	10. a (p. 342)	18. d (p. 349)	26. b (pp. 354-355)
3. a (p. 341)	11. c (p. 343)	19. b (p. 353)	27. c (p. 355)
4. e (p. 342)	12. c (p. 344)	20. d (p. 353)	28. d (p. 355)
5. a (p. 342)	13. a (p. 344)	21. d (p. 353)	29. a (pp. 354, 356)
6. a (p. 340)	14. b (p. 345)	22. c (p. 355)	30. e (pp. 355-356)
7. d (p. 340)	15. d (p. 347)	23. a (p. 353)	
8. b (p. 342)	16. c (p. 347)	24. b (p. 353)	

Short Answer Questions

1. require bile for digestion/absorption; travel in lymph initially within chylomicrons, and may require protein carriers for blood transport; stored primarily in liver and adipose tissue; pose a toxicity risk
2. vitamin A, vitamin D, vitamin E, vitamin K
3. promoting vision; participating in protein synthesis and cell differentiation; supporting reproduction and regulating growth
4. susceptibility to infectious diseases; night blindness; total blindness (xerophthalmia); keratinization
5. bone defects, birth defects
6. bone mineralization
7. rickets, osteomalacia, osteoporosis
8. fat-soluble antioxidant
9. erythrocyte hemolysis
10. synthesis of blood-clotting and bone proteins
11. fat malabsorption; use of certain drugs (antibiotics or anticoagulants)

Problem Solving

1. 7,930 IU × 0.05 µg RAE/IU = 396.5 µg RAE
   20,000 IU × 0.15 µg RAE/IU = 3,000 µg RAE

2. 3 oz. liver = 6,582 µg RAE; RDA for adult female = 700 µg RAE
   6,582 µg RAE divided by 3 = 2,194 µg RAE
   2,194 µg RAE divided by 700 µg RAE × 100% = 313%

✪ Chapter 12 – Water and the Major Minerals ✪

Chapter Outline

I. Water and the Body Fluids
   A. Water Balance and Recommended Intakes
      1. Water Intake
      2. Water Sources
      3. Water Losses
      4. Water Recommendations
      5. Health Effects of Water
   B. Blood Volume and Blood Pressure
      1. ADH
      2. Renin
      3. Angiotensin
      4. Aldosterone
   C. Fluid and Electrolyte Balance
      1. Dissociation of Salt in Water
      2. Electrolytes Attract Water
      3. Water Follows Electrolytes
      4. Proteins Regulate Flow of Fluids and Ions
      5. Regulation of Fluid and Electrolyte Balance
   D. Fluid and Electrolyte Imbalance
      1. Different Solutes Lost by Different Routes
      2. Replacing Lost Fluids and Electrolytes
   E. Acid-Base Balance
      1. Regulation by the Buffers
      2. Respiration in the Lungs
      3. Excretion in the Kidneys
II. The Minerals—An Overview
   A. Inorganic Elements
   B. The Body's Handling of Minerals
   C. Variable Bioavailability
   D. Nutrient Interactions
III. The Major Minerals
   A. Sodium
      1. Sodium Roles in the Body
      2. Sodium Recommendations
      3. Sodium and Hypertension
      4. Sodium and Bone Loss (Osteoporosis)
      5. Sodium in Foods
      6. Sodium Deficiency
      7. Sodium Toxicity and Excessive Intakes
   B. Chloride

      1. Chloride Roles in the Body
      2. Chloride Recommendations and Intakes
      3. Chloride Deficiency and Toxicity
   C. Potassium
      1. Potassium Roles in the Body
      2. Potassium Recommendations and Intakes
      3. Potassium and Hypertension
      4. Potassium Deficiency
      5. Potassium Toxicity
   D. Calcium
      1. Calcium Roles in the Body
      2. Calcium in Disease Prevention
      3. Calcium Balance
      4. Calcium Absorption
      5. Calcium Recommendations
      6. Calcium Food Sources
      7. Calcium Deficiency
   E. Phosphorus
      1. Phosphorus Roles in the Body
      2. Phosphorus Recommendations and Intakes
   F. Magnesium
      1. Magnesium Roles in the Body
      2. Magnesium Intakes
      3. Magnesium Deficiency
      4. Magnesium and Hypertension
      5. Magnesium Toxicity
   G. Sulfate
IV. Osteoporosis and Calcium
   A. Bone Development and Disintegration
   B. Age and Bone Calcium
      1. Maximizing Bone Mass
      2. Minimizing Bone Loss
   C. Gender and Hormones
   D. Genetics
   E. Physical Activity and Body Weight
   F. Smoking and Alcohol
   G. Dietary Calcium
   H. Other Nutrients
   I. A Perspective on Calcium Supplements
   J. Some Closing Thoughts

Summing Up

Water makes up about 1._____ percent of the adult body's weight. It assists with the 2._____ of nutrients and waste products throughout the body, participates in 3._____ reactions, acts as a 4._____, serves as a shock 5._____, and regulates body 6._____. To maintain water balance, intake from liquids, foods, and metabolism must equal 7._____ from the kidneys, skin, lungs, and GI tract. Whenever the body experiences 8._____ blood volume, low blood pressure, or highly concentrated body 9._____, the actions of ADH, renin, angiotensin, and 10._____ restore homeostasis. Electrolytes (charged minerals) in the fluids help 11._____ the fluids inside and outside the cells, thus ensuring the appropriate 12._____ balance and acid-base balance to support all life processes. Excessive losses of fluids and 13._____ upset these balances, and the kidneys play a key role in restoring 14._____.

Compared with the trace minerals, the major minerals are found, and needed, in 15._____ quantities in the body. Unlike vitamins and the energy-yielding nutrients, minerals are 16._____ elements that retain their chemical identities. Minerals usually receive special handling and 17._____ in the body, and they may bind with other substances or 18._____ with other minerals, thus limiting their 19._____.

Sodium is the main 20._____ outside cells and one of the primary electrolytes responsible for maintaining 21._____ balance. Dietary deficiency is unlikely, and excesses raise blood 22._____ in many people. For this reason, health professionals advise a diet 23._____ in salt and sodium.

Chloride is the major 24._____ outside cells, and it associates closely with sodium. In addition to its role in fluid balance, chloride is part of the stomach's 25._____ acid.

Potassium, like sodium and chloride, is an 26._____ that plays an important role in maintaining fluid balance. Potassium is the primary 27._____ inside cells; fresh foods, notably fruits and 28._____, are its best sources.

Most of the body's calcium is in the 29._____ where it provides a rigid structure and a reservoir of calcium for the blood. Blood calcium participates in muscle 30._____, blood clotting, and nerve impulses, and it is closely regulated by a system of 31._____ and vitamin D. Calcium is found predominantly in milk and milk products. Even when calcium intake is 32._____, blood calcium remains normal, but at the expense of 33._____ _____, which can lead to osteoporosis.

Phosphorus accompanies calcium both in the crystals of 34._____ and in many foods such as milk. Phosphorus is also important in 35._____ _____ as part of ATP, in lipid transport as part of 36._____, and in genetic materials as part of DNA and RNA.

Like calcium and phosphorus, magnesium supports 37._____ mineralization. Magnesium is also involved in numerous 38._____ systems and in heart function. It is found abundantly in 39._____ and dark green, leafy vegetables and, in some areas, in water.

Like the other nutrients, minerals' actions are 40._____ to get the body's work done. The 41._____ minerals, especially sodium, chloride, and potassium, influence the body's 42._____ _____; whenever an anion moves, a 43._____ moves—always maintaining homeostasis. Sodium, chloride, potassium, calcium, and magnesium are key members of the team of nutrients that direct 44._____ impulse transmission and muscle 45._____. They are also the primary nutrients involved in regulating blood 46._____. Phosphorus and magnesium participate in many reactions involving glucose, fatty acids, amino acids, and the 47._____. Calcium, phosphorus, and magnesium combine to form the structure of the bones and 48._____. Each major mineral also plays other specific roles in the body.

Chapter Study Questions

1. List the roles of water in the body.

2. List the sources of water intake and routes of water excretion.

3. What is ADH? Where does it exert its action? What is aldosterone? How does it work?

4. How does the body use electrolytes to regulate fluid balance?

5. What do the terms *major* and *trace* mean when describing the minerals in the body?

6. Describe some characteristics of minerals that distinguish them from vitamins.

7. What is the major function of sodium in the body? Describe how the kidneys regulate blood sodium. Is a dietary deficiency of sodium likely? Why or why not?

146

8. Describe the roles of chloride and conditions that may cause a chloride deficiency or toxicity.

9. List potassium's roles in the body and significant food sources of potassium.

10. List calcium's roles in the body. How does the body keep blood calcium constant regardless of intake?

11. Name significant food sources of calcium. What are the consequences of inadequate intakes?

12. List the roles of phosphorus in the body. Discuss the relationship between calcium and phosphorus. Is a dietary deficiency of phosphorus likely? Why or why not?

13. Identify the main roles, deficiency symptoms, and foods sources of magnesium.

14. Identify the main roles of sulfate and a condition that could cause a deficiency.

Key Terms Practice

To complete the crossword puzzle, identify the key term that best matches each definition.

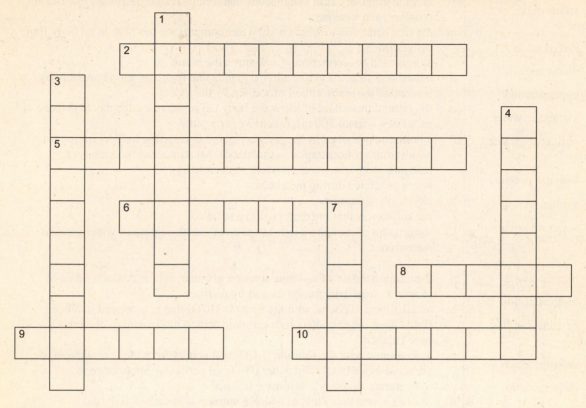

Across:

2. A hormone secreted by the thyroid gland that regulates blood calcium by lowering it when levels rise too high.
5. A disease in which the bones become porous and fragile due to a loss of minerals.
6. Chemical compounds in foods that combine with nutrients (especially minerals) to form complexes the body cannot absorb.
8. An enzyme from the kidneys that hydrolyzes the protein angiotensinogen to angiotensin I.
9. A mineral present in the body as part of some proteins.
10. A salt produced from the oxidation of sulfur.

Down:

1. A cation within the body's cells, active in many enzyme systems.
3. A major mineral found mostly in the body's bones and teeth.
4. The major anion in the extracellular fluids of the body.
7. The principal cation in the extracellular fluids of the body; critical to the maintenance of fluid balance, nerve impulse transmissions, and muscle contractions.

148

Match the key terms with their definitions.

11. _____ aldosterone

12. _____ antidiuretic hormone

13. _____ dehydration

14. _____ dissociates

15. _____ hyponatremia

16. _____ metabolic water

17. _____ obligatory water excretion

18. _____ osmotic pressure

19. _____ solutes

20. _____ water intoxication

a. the condition in which body water output exceeds water input; symptoms include thirst, dry skin and mucous membranes, rapid heartbeat, low blood pressure, and weakness

b. the rare condition in which body water contents are too high in all body fluid compartments

c. a decreased concentration of sodium in the blood

d. a hormone secreted by the adrenal glands that regulates blood pressure by increasing the reabsorption of sodium by the kidneys

e. the minimum amount of water the body has to excrete each day to dispose of its wastes—about 500 mL (about 2 c, or a pint)

f. a hormone produced by the pituitary gland in response to dehydration (or a high sodium concentration in the blood) that stimulates the kidneys to reabsorb more water and therefore to excrete less

g. water generated during metabolism

h. physically separates

i. the substances that are dissolved in a solution

j. the amount of pressure needed to prevent the movement of water across a membrane

21. _____ bicarbonate

22. _____ bioavailability

23. _____ calcium-binding protein

24. _____ calcium tetany

25. _____ carbonic acid

26. _____ mineralization

27. _____ oral rehydration therapy

28. _____ parathyroid hormone

29. _____ peak bone mass

30. _____ potassium

a. the administration of a simple solution of sugar, salt, and water, taken by mouth, to treat dehydration caused by diarrhea

b. an alkaline compound with the formula HCO_3 that is produced in all cell fluids from the dissociation of carbonic acid to help maintain the body's acid-base balance

c. a compound with the formula H_2CO_3 that results from the combination of carbon dioxide (CO_2) and water (H_2O); of particular importance in maintaining the body's acid-base balance

d. the rate at and the extent to which a nutrient is absorbed and used

e. the principal cation within the body's cells; critical to the maintenance of fluid balance, nerve impulse transmissions, and muscle contractions

f. the process in which calcium, phosphorus, and other minerals crystallize on the collagen matrix of a growing bone, hardening the bone

g. a hormone from the parathyroid glands that regulates blood calcium by raising it when levels fall too low

h. intermittent spasm of the extremities due to nervous and muscular excitability caused by low blood calcium concentrations

i. a protein in the intestinal cells, made with the help of vitamin D, that facilitates calcium absorption

j. the highest attainable bone density for an individual, developed during the first three decades of life

Sample Test Questions

Select the best answer for each question.

1. The most essential nutrient is:
   a. carbohydrate.
   b. protein.
   c. fat.
   d. water.

2. The percentage of water in the body is about:
   a. 20%.
   c. 60%.
   b. 40%.
   d. 90%.

3. The proportion of water is smaller in a person who is:
   a. male.
   b. muscular.
   c. obese.
   d. active.

4. Water is involved in all of the following **except**:
   a. regulation of body temperature.
   b. conversion of lipids to amino acids.
   c. shock absorption in the spinal cord.
   d. lubrication of joints.

5. People must have water in their diets because the:
   a. kidneys exert no control over the amount of water excreted in the urine.
   b. fluid lost from the body must be replaced.
   c. kidneys must excrete a minimum amount of water in the urine to rid the body of wastes.
   d. a and b
   e. b and c

6. Fluid within the cells is called:
   a. intracellular fluid.
   b. interstitial fluid.
   c. extracellular fluid.
   d. ionic fluid.

7. Among the following, the largest component of extracellular fluid is:
   a. intracellular fluid.
   b. interstitial fluid.
   c. electrolytes.
   d. ions.

8. Which of the following is false about dehydration?
   a. Water output exceeds water intake.
   b. Symptoms include thirst and dry skin.
   c. Symptoms include high blood pressure.
   d. Symptoms include rapid heartbeat and weakness.

9. The amount of water the body has to excrete each day to dispose of its wastes is:
   a. about 1500 mL.
   b. obligatory water excretion.
   c. insensible water losses.
   d. water intoxication.

10. The best water to drink for health reasons is:
    a. bottled water.
    b. carbonated water.
    c. soft water.
    d. hard water.

11. Which of the following substances is an electrolyte?
    a. Water
    b. Sodium
    c. A fatty acid
    d. Glucose
    e. Carbon

12. A cell membrane is an example of:
    a. a selectively permeable membrane.
    b. a water impermeable membrane.
    c. an anion.
    d. an electrolyte.

13. The amount and type of electrolytes in the body are largely regulated by:
    a. the liver.
    b. the kidneys.
    c. the intestines.
    d. the spleen.
    e. the pancreas.

14. Aldosterone secretion stimulates:
    a. sodium retention.
    b. sodium excretion.
    c. water excretion.
    d. a and c
    e. b and c

150

15. Buffers:
    a. move water into a concentrated solution.
    b. transport oxygen in the blood.
    c. maintain acid-base balance in the body.
    d. maintain blood pressure in the body.

16. Generally, the foods that have the highest sodium content are:
    a. fresh vegetables.
    b. canned fruits.
    c. roasted meats.
    d. processed foods.

17. The major anion of extracellular fluid is:
    a. sodium.
    b. calcium.
    c. potassium.
    d. sulfur.
    e. chloride.

18. People who respond to a high salt intake with an increase in blood pressure may have:
    a. dehydration.
    b. hypotension.
    c. salt cravings.
    d. salt sensitivity.

19. The *Dietary Guidelines* advise healthy Caucasians under 51 years of age to limit daily sodium intake to:
    a. <400 mg.
    b. <700 mg.
    c. <1500 mg.
    d. <2300 mg.

20. In cases of ultra-endurance competitive athletic events, athletes:
    a. should take salt tablets.
    b. may develop hyponatremia.
    c. are at risk for hypertension.
    d. should consume no more than 400 mg sodium per day.

21. The most reliable food source(s) of chloride is/are:
    a. meats and whole-grain cereals.
    b. salts and processed foods.
    c. dark green vegetables.
    d. public water.
    e. milk and milk products.

22. The richest food sources of potassium are:
    a. processed foods.
    b. ready-to-eat cereals.
    c. fresh foods of all kinds.
    d. cured meats.

23. Blood calcium levels can be increased by:
    1. better absorption of calcium in the intestines.
    2. retention of calcium by the kidneys.
    3. release of calcium from the bones.
    4. inhibition of osteoclast activity.
    5. release of calcium from the teeth.

    a. 1, 2
    b. 1, 2, 3
    c. 1, 2, 3, 5
    d. 3, 4

24. Factors that impair calcium absorption include:
    a. vitamin D.
    b. a high-fiber diet.
    c. phytates.
    d. a and b
    e. b and c

25. An inadequate intake of calcium for many years can lead to:
    a. osteoporosis.
    b. impaired energy-nutrient metabolism.
    c. pernicious anemia.
    d. bleeding gums and ease in bruising.
    e. peptic ulcers.

26. A class of foods that is rich in calcium and phosphorus is:
    a. citrus fruits.
    b. milk and milk products.
    c. starchy vegetables.
    d. root vegetables.
    e. liver and other organ meats.

27. Positive calcium balance is favored by:
    a. a high sodium intake.
    b. fiber.
    c. vitamin D.
    d. b and c

28. Phosphorus deficiencies are:
    a. rare.
    b. common.
    c. irreversible.
    d. a and b
    e. b and c

29. Magnesium:
    a. is directly necessary for protein synthesis in cells.
    b. protects bone structures against degeneration.
    c. is the body's principal intracellular electrolyte.
    d. is necessary for wound healing.
    e. helps maintain gastric acidity.

30. Sulfate:
    a. is found mainly in the adipose tissue.
    b. is commonly deficient.
    c. has an RDA of 400 mg.
    d. is present in rigid proteins.

Short Answer Questions

1. Three sources of water for the body are:

    a.

    b.

    c.

2. Four routes of water excretion are:

    a.

    b.

    c.

    d.

3. The seven major minerals are:

    a.

    b.

    c.

    d.

    e.

    f.

    g.

4. The six trace minerals are:

    a.

    b.

    c.

    d.

    e.

    f.

5. Two major minerals that are rarely lacking in American diets are:

    a.

    b.

152

6. Rich sources of potassium are:

   a.   c.

   b.

7. The two minerals that are most abundant in the body and found in bones and teeth are:

   a.   b.

8. Two minerals that are involved in protein building and stabilization are:

   a.   b.

Problem Solving

1. A sedentary 40-year-old male and a 27-year-old female professional basketball player each expend 2200 kcal per day. Calculate the water recommendation in cups based on energy expenditure for these two individuals.

2. How do the water recommendations you calculated in question #1 compare to the DRI recommendations?

3. Suppose that a soup recipe calls for 2 tsp of salt. How many grams of salt is that? How many grams of sodium are in that much salt?

4. If a cup of milk provides 300 mg of calcium and you are trying to consume 800 mg of calcium per day, how many cups of milk do you need to drink (assuming this is your only source of calcium)?

✆ Chapter 12 Answer Key ✇

Summing Up

1. 60
2. transport
3. chemical
4. solvent
5. absorber
6. temperature
7. losses
8. low
9. fluids
10. aldosterone
11. distribute
12. water
13. electrolytes
14. homeostasis
15. larger
16. inorganic
17. regulation
18. interact
19. absorption
20. cation
21. fluid
22. pressure
23. moderate
24. anion
25. hydrochloric
26. electrolyte
27. cation
28. vegetables
29. bones
30. contraction
31. hormones
32. inadequate
33. bone loss
34. bone
35. energy metabolism
36. phospholipids
37. bone
38. enzyme
39. legumes
40. coordinated
41. major
42. fluid balance
43. cation
44. nerve
45. contraction
46. pressure
47. vitamins
48. teeth

Chapter Study Questions

1. Water carries nutrients and waste products throughout the body; helps to form the structure of macromolecules; actively participates in chemical reactions; serves as the solvent for minerals, vitamins, amino acids, glucose, and many other small molecules; acts as a lubricant around joints; serves as shock absorber inside the eyes, the spinal cord, and the amniotic sac during pregnancy; aids in the body's temperature regulation; and maintains blood volume.

2. Sources of intake: liquids, foods, metabolic water. Routes of excretion: kidneys, skin, lungs, feces.

3. ADH is a hormone released by the pituitary gland in response to dehydration or high Na concentration in blood. It exerts its action on the kidneys, and they respond by reabsorbing water, thus preventing water loss. Aldosterone is a hormone secreted by the adrenal glands that stimulates the excretion of potassium and reabsorption of sodium by the kidneys. Since water follows sodium, this results in water retention and increased blood pressure.

4. The body uses electrolytes to control the movement of water inside cells and between cells. Since water is attracted to electrolytes and will follow them, the cells can induce water to flow across a membrane by moving electrolytes to the other side (creating a more concentrated solution on the target side).

5. Major minerals are needed in the largest amounts in the body (>100 mg/day); trace minerals are needed in small amounts in the body (<100 mg/day). Both are essential to life and health.

6. Minerals retain their chemical identity because they are inorganic elements rather than organic molecules made up of elements. Thus, they cannot be destroyed during food processing or preparation like vitamins. Their bioavailability may be influenced by the presence of binders, food compounds that combine with minerals to produce non-absorbable complexes.

7. Na's major function is to maintain fluid and electrolyte balance. The kidneys retain or excrete sodium and water to maintain appropriate sodium concentrations and regulate blood pressure. A dietary deficiency of sodium is not likely because of sodium's abundance in food products.

8. Chloride helps maintain fluid and electrolyte balance. In the stomach, the chloride ion is part of hydrochloric acid, which maintains the strong acidity of the gastric juice. Chloride losses may occur in conditions such as heavy sweating, chronic diarrhea, and vomiting. One of the most serious consequences of vomiting is the loss of hydrochloric acid from the stomach, which upsets the acid-base balance. The only known cause of elevated blood chloride concentrations is dehydration due to water deficiency. In both cases, consuming ordinary foods and beverages can restore chloride balance.

9. Potassium plays a major role in maintaining fluid and electrolyte balance and cell integrity. During nerve impulse transmissions and muscle contractions, potassium and sodium briefly trade places across the cell

membrane. The cell then quickly pumps them back into place. Controlling potassium distribution is a high priority for the body because it affects many aspects of homeostasis, including a steady heartbeat. Because cells remain intact unless foods are processed, the richest sources of potassium are fresh foods. Potassium is found in all food groups, notably vegetables, fruits, and milk and milk products.

10. Ca's roles: maintains bone and tooth structure, helps regulate blood pressure, participates in blood clotting, and binds to and activates cell proteins involved in regulation of muscle contractions, nerve impulse transmission, hormone secretion, and enzyme reaction activation. When levels fall, intestinal absorption increases, bone withdrawal increases, and kidney excretion diminishes; these processes are regulated by parathyroid hormone and vitamin D. When blood levels of calcium rise, calcitonin is secreted. Calcitonin inhibits the activation of vitamin D, prevents calcium reabsorption in the kidneys, limits calcium absorption in the intestines, and inhibits osteoclast cells from breaking down bone, preventing the release of calcium.

11. Calcium is found predominantly in milk and milk products. Inadequate intakes limit the bones' ability to achieve optimal mass and density and increase risk of osteoporosis and associated fractures.

12. P's roles: part of bone structure, part of DNA and RNA, activates enzymes, part of ATP, and part of phospholipid structure and cell membranes. Ca and P combine within the hydroxyapatite crystals of bone and teeth, providing strength and rigidity. A deficiency is unlikely because phosphorus is commonly found in almost all foods; it is especially abundant in animal tissues, eggs, and milk.

13. In addition to maintaining bone health, magnesium acts in all the cells of the soft tissues, where it forms part of the protein-making machinery and is necessary for energy metabolism. It participates in hundreds of enzyme systems; it is essential to the body's use of glucose; the synthesis of protein, fat, and nucleic acids; and the cells' membrane transport systems. It is involved in muscle contraction (a severe deficiency causes tetany) and blood clotting. Magnesium supports the normal functioning of the immune system. Low magnesium intake may upset bone metabolism and increase the risk for osteoporosis. Magnesium deficiency may exacerbate inflammation and contribute to chronic diseases such as heart disease, hypertension, diabetes, and cancer. Magnesium deficiencies also impair central nervous system activity and may be responsible for the hallucinations experienced during alcohol withdrawal. Magnesium is critical to heart function and seems to protect against hypertension and heart disease. Magnesium is found abundantly in legumes and leafy green vegetables and, in some areas, in water.

14. Sulfate is involved in stabilization of the protein structure. Because the body's sulfate needs are easily met with normal protein intakes, there is no recommended intake for sulfate. Deficiencies do not occur when diets contain protein. Only when people lack protein to the point of severe deficiency will they lack the sulfur-containing amino acids.

Key Terms Practice

1. magnesium
2. calcitonin
3. phosphorus
4. chloride
5. osteoporosis
6. binders
7. sodium
8. renin
9. sulfur
10. sulfate
11. d
12. f
13. a
14. h
15. c
16. g
17. e
18. j
19. i
20. b
21. b
22. d
23. i
24. h
25. c
26. f
27. a
28. g
29. j
30. e

Sample Test Questions

1. d (p. 367)
2. c (p. 368)
3. c (p. 368)
4. b (p. 368)
5. e (p. 369)
6. a (p. 368)
7. b (p. 368)
8. c (p. 368-369)
9. b (p. 369)
10. d (p. 370)
11. b (p. 373)
12. a (p. 374)
13. b (pp. 375, 377)
14. a (p. 372)
15. c (p. 377)
16. d (p. 381)
17. e (p. 382)
18. d (p. 379)
19. d (p. 380)
20. b (p. 381)
21. b (p. 382)
22. c (p. 383)
23. b (pp. 385-386)
24. e (p. 386)
25. a (pp. 388-389)
26. b (pp. 387, 390)
27. c (p. 386)
28. a (p. 390)

29. a (p. 392)   30. d (p. 393)

Short Answer Questions

1.   beverages, foods, metabolic water (water released during energy metabolism)

2.   kidneys (urine), lungs (exhaled vapor), skin (sweat), feces

3.   sodium, chloride, potassium, calcium, phosphorus, magnesium, sulfur (sulfate)

4.   iron, zinc, copper, manganese, iodine, selenium

5.   sodium, chloride

6.   vegetables, fruits, milk and milk products

7.   calcium, phosphorus

8.   magnesium, sulfate

Problem Solving

1.   Sedentary male: 1.0-1.5 mL/kcal × 2200 kcal = 2200-3300 mL/day × 0.5 c/125 mL = 8.8-13.2 c
     Female athlete: 1.5 mL/kcal × 2200 kcal = 3300 mL/day × 0.5 c/125 mL = 13.2 c

2.   2200-3300 mL/day × 1 L/1000 mL = 2.2-3.3 L/day; 3300 mL/day × 1 L/1000 mL = 3.3 L/day
     The AI for total water are 3.7 L/day for an adult male and 2.7 L/day for an adult female. The calculated
     recommendation of 2.2-3.3 L/day for the sedentary male is somewhat lower than the AI, whereas the calculated
     recommendation of 3.3 L/day for the female athlete is significantly higher. This seems reasonable since water
     losses via sweat would be expected to be greater in a female athlete than in the average adult female.

3.   2 tsp × 6 g/tsp =   12 g salt
     2 tsp salt × 2300 mg Na/tsp = 4600 mg Na = 4.6 g sodium   OR   12 g salt × 40% = 4.8 g sodium

4.   800 mg divided by 300 mg/c = 2.7 c

❧ Chapter 13 – The Trace Minerals ❧

Chapter Outline

I.   The Trace Minerals—An Overview
   A.   Food Sources
   B.   Deficiencies
   C.   Toxicities
   D.   Interactions
   E.   Nonessential Trace Minerals
II. The Trace Minerals
   A.   Iron
      1.   Iron Roles in the Body
      2.   Iron Absorption
      3.   Iron Transport and Storage
      4.   Iron Deficiency
      5.   Assessment of Iron Deficiency
      6.   Iron Deficiency and Anemia
      7.   Iron Deficiency and Behavior
      8.   Iron Deficiency and Pica
      9.   Iron Overload
     10. Iron and Chronic Disease
     11. Iron Poisoning
     12. Iron Recommendations
     13. Iron Food Sources
     14. Iron Contamination
     15. Iron Supplementation
   B.   Zinc
      1.   Zinc Roles in the Body
      2.   Zinc Absorption
      3.   Zinc Transport
      4.   Zinc Deficiency
      5.   Zinc Toxicity
      6.   Zinc Recommendations and Sources
      7.   Zinc Supplementation
   C.   Iodine
      1.   Iodide Roles in the Body
      2.   Iodine Deficiency
      3.   Iodine Toxicity
      4.   Iodine Recommendations and Sources
   D.   Selenium

      1.   Selenium Roles in the Body
      2.   Selenium Deficiency
      3.   Selenium and Cancer
      4.   Selenium Recommendations and
         Sources
      5.   Selenium Toxicity
   E.   Copper
      1.   Copper Roles in the Body
      2.   Copper Deficiency and Toxicity
      3.   Copper Recommendations and Sources
   F.   Manganese
      1.   Manganese Roles in the Body
      2.   Manganese Deficiency and Toxicity
      3.   Manganese Recommendations and
         Sources
   G.   Fluoride
      1.   Fluoride Roles in the Body
      2.   Fluoride Toxicity
      3.   Fluoride Recommendations and Sources
   H.   Chromium
      1.   Chromium Roles in the Body
      2.   Chromium Recommendations and
         Sources
      3.   Chromium Supplements
   I.   Molybdenum
III. Contaminant Minerals
IV. Phytochemicals and Functional Foods
   A.   The Phytochemicals
      1.   Defending against Cancer
      2.   Defending against Heart Disease
      3.   Defending against Other Diseases
      4.   The Phytochemicals in Perspective
   B.   Functional Foods
      1.   Foods as Pharmacy
      2.   Unanswered Questions
   C.   Future Foods

Summing Up

Although the body uses only tiny amounts of the trace minerals, they are 1._____ to health. Because so little is required, the trace minerals can be 2._____ at levels not far above estimated requirements—a consideration for 3._____ users. Like the other nutrients, the trace minerals are best obtained by eating a variety of 4._____ .

Most of the body's iron is in hemoglobin and 5._____, where it carries oxygen for use in energy metabolism; some iron is also required for 6._____ involved in a variety of reactions. Special proteins assist with iron absorption, 7._____, and storage—all helping to maintain an appropriate balance—

because both too little and too much iron can be 8._____. Iron deficiency is most common among infants and young children, teenagers, women of childbearing age, and 9._____ women. Symptoms include 10._____ and anemia. Iron overload is most common in 11._____. Heme iron, which is found only in meat, fish, and poultry, is better absorbed than 12._____ iron, which occurs in most foods. Nonheme iron absorption is improved by eating iron-containing foods with foods containing the MFP factor and 13._____ ___; absorption is limited by phytates and 14._____.

Zinc-requiring enzymes participate in a multitude of reactions affecting 15._____, vitamin A activity, and pancreatic digestive enzyme synthesis, among others. After a meal, both dietary zinc and zinc-rich pancreatic secretions (via 16._____ circulation) are absorbed. Absorption is regulated by a special binding protein (17._____) in the small intestine. Protein-rich foods derived from animals are the best sources of 18._____ zinc. Fiber and phytates in cereals bind zinc, limiting 19._____. Growth retardation and sexual 20._____ are hallmark symptoms of zinc deficiency.

Iodide, the ion of the mineral iodine, is an essential component of the 21._____ hormones. An iodine deficiency can lead to simple 22._____ (enlargement of the thyroid gland) and can impair fetal development, causing 23._____. Iodization of salt has largely eliminated iodine 24._____ in the United States and Canada.

Selenium is an antioxidant nutrient that works closely with the 25._____ _____ enzyme and vitamin E. Selenium is found in association with 26._____ in foods. Deficiencies are associated with a predisposition to a type of heart abnormality known as 27._____ disease.

Copper is a component of several enzymes, all of which are involved in some way with oxygen or 28._____. Some act as antioxidants; others are essential to 29._____ metabolism. Legumes, whole grains, and 30._____ are good sources of copper.

Manganese-dependent enzymes are involved in bone formation and various 31._____ processes. Because manganese is widespread in plant foods, 32._____ are rare, although regular use of calcium and iron supplements may limit manganese 33._____.

Fluoride makes bones stronger and teeth more resistant to 34._____. Fluoridation of public water supplies can significantly reduce the incidence of 35._____ _____, but excess fluoride during tooth development can cause 36._____—discolored and pitted tooth enamel.

Chromium enhances 37._____ action. A deficiency can impair glucose 38._____. Chromium is widely available in unrefined foods including brewer's yeast, whole grains, and 39._____.

Molybdenum is found in a variety of foods and participates in several 40._____ reactions.

Lead typifies the ways all heavy metals behave in the body: they interfere with 41._____ that are trying to do their jobs. The "good guy" nutrients are shoved aside by the "bad guy" 42._____. Then, when the contaminants cannot perform the roles of the nutrients, health

43._____. To safeguard our health, we must defend ourselves against

44._____ by eating nutrient-rich foods and preserving a clean environment.

Chapter Study Questions

1.   Summarize key factors unique to the trace minerals.

2.   Distinguish between heme and nonheme iron. Discuss the factors that enhance iron absorption.

3.   Distinguish between iron deficiency and iron-deficiency anemia. What are the symptoms of iron-deficiency anemia?

4.   What causes iron overload? What are its symptoms?

5.   Describe the similarities and differences in the absorption and regulation of iron and zinc.

6.   Discuss possible reasons for a low intake of zinc. What factors affect the bioavailability of zinc?

7.   Describe the principal functions of iodide, selenium, copper, manganese, fluoride, chromium, and molybdenum in the body.

8.   What public health measure has been used in preventing simple goiter? What measure has been recommended for protection against tooth decay?

9. Discuss the importance of a balanced and varied diet in obtaining the essential minerals and avoiding toxicities.

10. Describe some of the ways trace minerals interact with each other and with other nutrients.

11. Describe how contaminant minerals disrupt body processes and impair nutrition status.

Key Terms Practice

To complete the crossword puzzle, identify the key term that best matches each definition.

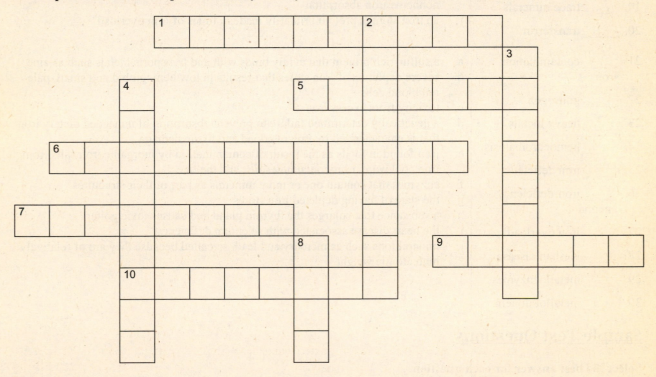

Across:
1. The percentage of total blood volume that consists of red blood cells.
5. A substance that can grasp the positive ions of a mineral.
6. The stabilized form of bone and tooth crystal, in which fluoride has replaced the hydroxyl groups of hydroxyapatite.
7. The iron storage protein.
9. An enlargement of the thyroid gland due to an iodine deficiency, malfunction of the gland, or overconsumption of a goitrogen.
10. A trace element.

Down:

2. A congenital disease characterized by mental and physical retardation and commonly caused by maternal iodine deficiency during pregnancy.
3. A hormone produced by the liver that regulates iron balance.
4. Discoloration and pitting of tooth enamel caused by excess fluoride during tooth development.
8. A craving for and consumption of nonfood substances.

Match the key terms with their definitions.

11. _____ bioavailability
12. _____ cofactor
13. _____ heme iron
14. _____ hemoglobin
15. _____ hemosiderin
16. _____ MFP factor
17. _____ myoglobin
18. _____ nonheme iron
19. _____ trace minerals
20. _____ transferrin

a. essential mineral nutrients the human body requires in relatively small amounts (less than 100 milligrams per day)
b. the rate at and the extent to which a nutrient is absorbed and used
c. a substance that works with an enzyme to facilitate a chemical reaction
d. the oxygen-carrying protein of the red blood cells that transports oxygen from the lungs to tissues throughout the body
e. the oxygen-holding protein of the muscle cells
f. the iron transport protein
g. the iron in foods that is bound proteins; found only in meat, fish, and poultry
h. the iron in foods that is not bound to proteins; found in both plant-derived and animal-derived foods
i. a peptide released during the digestion of meat, fish, and poultry that enhances nonheme iron absorption
j. an iron storage protein primarily made in times of iron overload

21. _____ contamination iron
22. _____ goitrogen
23. _____ heavy metals
24. _____ hemochromatosis
25. _____ iron deficiency
26. _____ iron-deficiency anemia
27. _____ iron overload
28. _____ Keshan disease
29. _____ metalloenzymes
30. _____ metallothionein

a. a sulfur-rich protein that avidly binds with and transports metals such as zinc
b. severe depletion of iron stores that results in low hemoglobin and small, pale red blood cells
c. toxicity from excess iron
d. a genetically determined failure to prevent absorption of unneeded dietary iron that is characterized by iron overload and tissue damage
e. iron found in foods as the result of contamination by inorganic iron salts from iron cookware, iron-containing soils, and the like
f. enzymes that contain one or more minerals as part of their structures
g. the state of having depleted iron stores
h. a substance that enlarges the thyroid gland and causes toxic goiter
i. the heart disease associated with selenium deficiency
j. mineral ions such as mercury and lead, so called because they are of relatively high atomic weight

Sample Test Questions

Select the best answer for each question.

1. Essential mineral nutrients that the human body requires in small amounts (<100 mg/day) are called:
   a. macrominerals.
   b. major minerals.
   c. trace minerals.
   d. minor minerals.

2. Which of the following is true about microminerals?
   a. The body requires them in large amounts.
   b. They participate in specific tasks only in one area of the body.
   c. The micromineral contents of foods are unaffected by soil composition.
   d. Factors in the diet and within the body affect the bioavailability of minerals.

3. The most common result of a trace mineral deficiency in children is:
    a. GI tract problems.
    b. failure to grow and thrive.
    c. problems with muscles.
    d. central nervous system failure.

4. Since toxicities can easily develop at intakes of trace minerals not far above the requirements,
    a. the supplement industry prepares products below the recommendations.
    b. the FDA requires that amounts of trace minerals in supplements be limited.
    c. consumers must be aware of possible dangers and select supplements carefully.
    d. a and b
    e. a and c

5. Which of the following statements is true about interactions among the trace minerals?
    a. Interactions are uncommon and unnecessary.
    b. Interactions may lead to nutrient imbalances.
    c. Taking high doses of supplements benefits interactions of trace minerals.
    d. a and b
    e. b and c

6. Iron is important in the body because it is:
    a. needed for blood clotting.
    b. an integral part of bones and teeth.
    c. a constituent of hemoglobin.
    d. an antioxidant.

7. Which of the following iron-containing compounds transports iron from the intestine to the liver and bone marrow?
    a. Ferritin
    b. Myoglobin
    c. Transferrin
    d. Hemoglobin

8. The most common symptom of an iron deficiency is:
    a. night blindness.
    b. abnormal blood clotting.
    c. anemia.
    d. a skin rash.
    e. hemophilia.

9. Pica is:
    a. an appetite for ice, clay, paste, or other nonfood substances.
    b. a mineral deficiency associated with a certain area of the country.
    c. a localized skin rash.
    d. a cancer-causing additive.

10. The hemoglobin level in the blood is used to assess a person's _____ status.
    a. copper
    b. folate
    c. vitamin B_{12}
    d. iron
    e. zinc

11. The iron-storage protein made in times of iron overload is:
    a. myoglobin.
    b. hemosiderin.
    c. heme.
    d. transferrin.

12. The measurement of the volume of red blood cells packed in a given volume of blood is:
    a. ferritin.
    b. hepcidin.
    c. hematocrit.
    d. heme.

13. Which of the following is characterized by iron overload and tissue damage?
    a. Hemochromatosis
    b. Menkes disease
    c. High erythrocyte protoporphyrin
    d. Hemosiderosis

14. People at high risk for iron deficiency include:
    a. older men and women.
    b. middle-aged men.
    c. infants and young children.
    d. All of the above

15. Which foods contribute the most iron per stated portion?
    a. Meats, fish, and poultry (3 oz.)
    b. Milk (1 cup)
    c. Carrots and green beans (1 cup)
    d. Peaches and pears (1 cup)

16. A very poor source of iron is:
    a. legumes.
    b. dried fruits.
    c. whole-grain breads.
    d. milk.

17. An important function of zinc is to support the work of:
    a. DNA.
    b. metalloenzymes.
    c. protein carriers.
    d. oxygen carriers.

18. Zinc is involved in the circulatory route from the pancreas to the intestine and back to the pancreas. This is called:
    a. enterohepatic circulation.
    b. oxalate-bound transport.
    c. ligand-operating absorption.
    d. cofactor assistance.
    e. enteropancreatic circulation.

19. Which of the following is **not** a zinc deficiency symptom?
    a. Severe growth retardation
    b. Arrested sexual maturation
    c. Decreased taste sensitivity
    d. Pernicious anemia

20. Among the following, the best sources of available zinc are:
    a. shellfish, meats, and poultry.
    b. breads, cereals, and grains.
    c. fruits and vegetables.
    d. milk products.

21. Which of the following statements is true about zinc supplementation?
    a. People in developed countries should take zinc supplements.
    b. Zinc lozenges are effective at reducing incidence of the common cold.
    c. Zinc lozenges have no side effects.
    d. In developing countries, zinc supplements play a major role in treatment of childhood infectious diseases.

22. Consumption of which of the following would best help to ensure normal iodide intake?
    a. Liver
    b. Irradiated milk
    c. Salt-water fish
    d. Fortified margarine

23. Cretinism is caused by a deficiency of:
    a. copper.
    b. iron.
    c. fluoride.
    d. zinc.
    e. iodide.

24. One of copper's roles is to:
    a. function as part of antioxidant enzymes.
    b. help manufacture collagen.
    c. assist in oxidation of ferrous iron to ferric iron.
    d. a and b
    e. a, b, and c

25. Which of the following statements is true about manganese?
    a. Manganese deficiencies are common in children.
    b. Manganese requirements are high.
    c. High intakes of calcium and iron limit manganese absorption.
    d. Manganese is found most in meat products.

26. Fluoride is necessary nutritionally for:
    a. hardness of the bones and teeth.
    b. production of the thyroid hormone.
    c. prevention of anemia.
    d. the metabolism of glucose.
    e. a and b

27. Excess fluoride can cause:
    a. deposition of calcium in soft tissues.
    b. a drastic increase in tooth decay.
    c. fluorosis.
    d. osteomalacia.

28. Selenium is involved in:
    a. hormone production.
    b. protein synthesis.
    c. antioxidant activities.
    d. glycogen breakdown.

29. Contaminant minerals impair the body's growth and work capacity. They:
    a. enter the food supply by way of soil, water, and air pollution.
    b. include lead and mercury.
    c. are food additives.
    d. a and b
    e. a, b and c

30. Cobalt seems to be important in nutrition as part of:
    a. vitamin A.
    b. glutathione peroxidase.
    c. vitamin B_{12}.
    d. vitamin B_6.

Short Answer Questions

1. The essential trace minerals are:
    a.   d.   g.
    b.   e.   h.
    c.   f.   i.

2. Iron's two ionic states are:
    a.   b.

3. Life-stage groups that are especially vulnerable to iron deficiency are:
    a.   c.
    b.   d.

4. Symptoms of hemochromatosis are:
    a.   c.
    b.

5. Absorption of nonheme iron is limited by:
    a.   c.
    b.   d.

164

6. Absorption of zinc is hindered by:

    a.   b.

7. Two major consequences of zinc deficiency in children are:

    a.   b.

8. Two serious conditions caused by iodine deficiency are:

    a.   b.

9. Roles of selenium-containing enzymes include:

    a.   b.

10. Two rare genetic disorders that affect copper status are:

    a.   b.

11. Copper is part of enzymes that:

    a.

    b.

12. Manganese-dependent enzymes are involved in:

    a.

    b.

    c.

13. Fluoride functions to:

    a.

    b.

14. Symptoms of a chromium deficiency may include:

    a.   c.

    b.   d.

15. Molybdenum-rich foods include:

    a.   d.

    b.   e.

    c.

16. Contaminant minerals known as heavy metals include:

    a.   c.

    b.

ꙮ Chapter 13 Answer Key ꙮ

Summing Up

1. vital
2. toxic
3. supplement
4. foods
5. myoglobin
6. enzymes
7. transport
8. damaging
9. pregnant
10. fatigue
11. men
12. nonheme

13. vitamin C
14. oxalates
15. growth
16. enteropancreatic
17. metallothionein
18. bioavailable
19. absorption
20. immaturity
21. thyroid
22. goiter
23. cretinism
24. deficiency

25. glutathione
    peroxidase
26. protein
27. Keshan
28. oxidation
29. iron
30. shellfish
31. metabolic
32. deficiencies
33. absorption
34. decay
35. dental caries

36. fluorosis
37. insulin's
38. homeostasis
39. liver
40. metabolic
41. nutrients
42. contaminants
43. diminishes
44. contamination

Chapter Study Questions

1. Although the body uses only tiny amounts of the trace minerals, they are vital to health. Because so little is required, the trace minerals can be toxic at levels not far above estimated requirements—a consideration for supplement users. Like the other nutrients, the trace minerals are best obtained by eating a variety of foods.

2. Heme iron is iron in foods that is bound to hemoglobin or myoglobin, and hence is only found in foods made from animal flesh. It is better absorbed than non-heme iron, which is not bound to proteins and is found in both plant- and animal-derived foods. Vitamin C, citric and lactic acids, sugars (fructose), and MFP factor enhance iron absorption.

3. Iron deficiency is the state of having depleted iron stores; iron-deficiency anemia is a condition of small and pale blood cells resulting from an iron deficiency that causes pallor, fatigue, weakness, headaches, apathy, and poor resistance to cold temperatures.

4. Iron overload is usually caused by a genetic failure to prevent unneeded iron absorption (hemochromatosis). The absence or ineffectiveness of the hormone hepcidin has been implicated. Less common causes include repeated blood transfusions, large doses of supplemental iron, and other metabolic disorders. Symptoms: fatigue, apathy, lethargy, free-radical tissue damage (especially to the liver), infections.

5. Similarities exist in absorption and regulation: absorption of both is partially determined by a person's status; other dietary factors can inhibit or facilitate absorption. Both are recycled within the body to a significant extent. Differences exist in that the intestine receives zinc from both ingested food and zinc-rich pancreatic secretions; the storage methods for each vary.

6. Diets very low in animal protein may be inadequate in zinc. Phytates and fiber inhibit absorption.

7. Iodide: part of thyroid hormones. Selenium: part of an enzyme that acts as an antioxidant, regulates thyroid hormone. Copper: part of enzymes, catalyst in hemoglobin formation, collagen synthesis. Manganese: acts as a cofactor for many enzymes that facilitate the metabolism of carbohydrate, lipids, and amino acids. Fluoride: part of crystal structure of bones and teeth. Chromium: enhances insulin action. Molybdenum: acts as a working part of several metalloenzymes.

8. Iodization of salt. Fluoridation of water.

9. Such a diet prevents an excess of one trace mineral from causing a deficiency of another, prevents a deficiency of one mineral that may cause a toxic reaction of another, provides factors that promote trace mineral absorption, and includes food sources that contain all the trace minerals.

10. Calcium and phytates inhibit nonheme iron absorption. Fiber and phytates bind zinc, limiting its bioavailability. Large doses of zinc inhibit iron and copper absorption. Vitamin C enhances nonheme iron absorption.

11. Lead typifies the ways all heavy metals behave in the body: they interfere with nutrients that are trying to do their jobs. A contaminant mineral is able to displace essential minerals from metabolic sites they normally occupy because it is chemically similar. However, because the contaminants cannot perform the roles of the nutrients, body functions are impaired and health diminishes.

Key Terms Practice

1.	hematocrit	9.	goiter	17.	e	25.	g
2.	cretinism	10.	selenium	18.	h	26.	b
3.	hepcidin	11.	b	19.	a	27.	c
4.	fluorosis	12.	c	20.	f	28.	i
5.	chelate	13.	g	21.	e	29.	f
6.	fluorapatite:	14.	d	22.	h	30.	a
7.	ferritin	15.	j	23.	j		
8.	pica	16.	i	24.	d		

Sample Test Questions

1.	c (p. 403)	9.	a (p. 410)	17.	b (pp. 414-415)	25.	c (p. 421)
2.	d (pp. 403-404)	10.	d (p. 409)	18.	e (p. 415)	26.	a (p. 422)
3.	b (p. 404)	11.	b (p. 407)	19.	d (p. 416)	27.	c (p. 422)
4.	c (p. 404)	12.	c (p. 409)	20.	a (p. 416)	28.	c (p. 419)
5.	b (p. 405)	13.	a (p. 411)	21.	d (p. 416)	29.	d (p. 424)
6.	c (p. 406)	14.	c (p. 409)	22.	c (p. 418)	30.	c (p. 405)
7.	c (pp. 406, 407)	15.	a (p. 413)	23.	e (p. 418)		
8.	c (p. 408)	16.	d (p. 413)	24.	e (p. 420)		

Short Answer Questions

1. iron, zinc, iodine, selenium, copper, manganese, fluoride, chromium, molybdenum

2. ferrous (reduced, Fe^{++}); ferric (oxidized, Fe^{+++})

3. women in reproductive years, pregnant women, infants and young children, adolescents

4. apathy, lethargy, fatigue

5. phytates, vegetable proteins, calcium, tannic acid

6. fiber, phytates

7. growth retardation, delayed sexual maturation

8. goiter, cretinism

9. defending against oxidation (antioxidants), regulation of thyroid hormones

10. Menkes diseases, Wilson's disease

11. catalyze the oxidation of ferrous iron to ferric iron (and thus are essential to iron metabolism), serve an antioxidant function

12. energy nutrient metabolism, bone formation, conversion of pyruvate to a TCA cycle compound

13. maintain health of bones and teeth, make teeth more resistant to decay

14. elevated blood glucose, impaired glucose tolerance, impaired insulin response, impaired glucagon response

15. legumes, breads and other grains, leafy green vegetables, milk, liver

16. lead, mercury, cadmium

⚲ Chapter 14 – Fitness: ⚲
Physical Activity, Nutrients, and Body Adaptations

Chapter Outline

I.   Fitness
   A. Benefits of Fitness
   B. Developing Fitness
      1. The Overload Principle
      2. The Body's Response to Physical Activity
      3. Cautions on Starting a Fitness Program
   C. Cardiorespiratory Endurance
      1. Cardiorespiratory Conditioning
      2. Muscle Conditioning
      3. A Balanced Fitness Program
   D. Resistance Training
II. Energy Systems and Fuels to Support Activity
   A. The Energy Systems of Physical Activity— ATP and CP
      1. ATP
      2. CP
      3. The Energy-Yielding Nutrients
   B. Glucose Use during Physical Activity
      1. Diet Affects Glycogen Storage and Use
      2. Intensity of Activity Affects Glycogen Use
      3. Lactate
      4. Duration of Activity Affects Glycogen Use
      5. Glucose Depletion
      6. Glucose during Activity
      7. Glucose after Activity
      8. Training Affects Glycogen Use
   C. Fat Use during Physical Activity
      1. Duration of Activity Affects Fat Use
      2. Intensity of Activity Affects Fat Use
      3. Training Affects Fat Use
   D. Protein Use during Physical Activity—and between Times
      1. Protein Used in Muscle Building
      2. Protein Used as Fuel
      3. Diet Affects Protein Use during Activity
      4. Intensity and Duration of Activity Affect Protein Use during Activity
      5. Training Affects Protein Use
      6. Protein Recommendations for Active People
III. Vitamins and Minerals to Support Activity
   A. Dietary Supplements
   B. Nutrients of Concern
      1. Vitamin E
      2. Iron Deficiency

      3. Iron-Deficiency Anemia
      4. Sports Anemia
      5. Iron Recommendations for Athletes
IV. Fluids and Electrolytes to Support Activity
   A. Temperature Regulation
      1. Hyperthermia
      2. Hypothermia
      3. Fluid Replacement via Hydration
      4. Electrolyte Losses and Replacement
      5. Hyponatremia
   B. Sports Drinks
      1. Fluid
      2. Glucose
      3. Sodium and Other Electrolytes
      4. Good Taste
      5. Enhanced Water
   C. Poor Beverage Choices: Caffeine and Alcohol
      1. Caffeine
      2. Alcohol
V. Diets for Physically Active People
   A. Choosing a Diet to Support Fitness
      1. Water
      2. Nutrient Density
      3. Carbohydrate
      4. Protein
   B. Meals before and after Competition
      1. Pregame Meals
      2. Postgame Meals
VI. Supplements as Ergogenic Aids
   A. Dietary Supplements that Perform as Claimed
      1. Convenient Dietary Supplements
      2. Caffeine
      3. Creatine
      4. Sodium Bicarbonate
   B. Dietary Supplements that May Perform as Claimed
      1. Beta-hydroxymethylbutyrate
      2. Ribose
   C. Dietary Supplements that Do Not Perform as Claimed
      1. Carnitine
      2. Chromium Picolinate
   D. Dangerous, Banned, or Illegal Supplements
      1. Anabolic Steroids
      2. DHEA and Androstenedione
      3. Human Growth Hormone

168

Summing Up

Physical activity brings good health and 1._____ life. To develop fitness—whose components are flexibility, muscle strength and endurance, and 2._____

_____—a person must condition the body, through training, to 3._____ to the activity performed.

The mixture of fuels the muscles use during physical activity depends on diet, the 4._____ and duration of the activity, and training. During intense activity, the fuel mix contains mostly 5._____, whereas during less intense, moderate activity, 6._____ makes a greater contribution. With endurance training, muscle cells adapt to store more 7._____ and to rely less on glucose and more on 8._____ for energy. Athletes in training may need more 9._____ than sedentary people do, but they typically eat more food as well and therefore obtain enough protein without 10._____.

With the possible exception of iron, well-nourished active people and athletes do not need nutrient 11._____. Women and teens may need to pay special attention to their 12._____ needs.

Active people need to drink plenty of 13._____; endurance athletes need to drink both water and 14._____-containing beverages, especially during training and competition. During events lasting longer than 15.____ hours, athletes need to pay special attention to replace sodium losses to prevent 16._____.

The person who wants to excel physically will apply accurate nutrition knowledge along with dedication to rigorous 17._____. A diet that provides ample fluid and includes a variety of 18._____-_____ foods in quantities to meet 19._____ needs will enhance not only athletic performance, but overall 20._____ as well. Carbohydrate-rich foods that are light and easy to digest are recommended for both the 21._____ and the postgame meal.

Chapter Study Questions

1. Define fitness, and list its benefits.

2. Explain the overload principle.

3. Define cardiorespiratory endurance and list some of its benefits.

4. What types of exercise are aerobic? Which are anaerobic?

5. Describe the relationships among energy expenditure, type of activity, and oxygen use.

6. What factors influence the body's use of glucose during physical activity? How?

7. What factors influence the body's use of fat during physical activity? How?

8. What factors influence the body's use of protein during physical activity? How?

9. Why are some athletes likely to develop iron-deficiency anemia? Compare iron-deficiency anemia and sports anemia, explaining the differences.

10. Discuss the importance of hydration during training, and list recommendations to maintain fluid balance.

11. Describe the components of a healthy diet for athletic performance.

Key Terms Practice

To complete the crossword puzzle, identify the key term that best matches each definition.

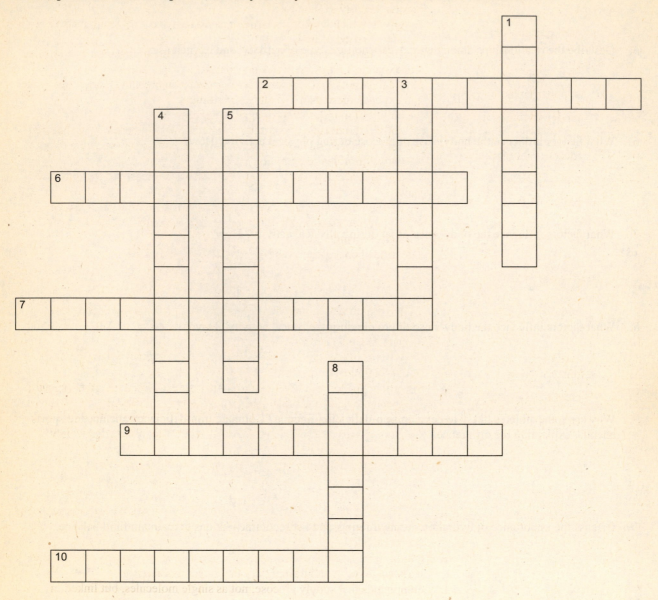

Across:
2. A below-normal body temperature.
6. An above-normal body temperature.
7. The physical effect of training; improved flexibility, strength, and endurance.
9. Growing larger; with regard to muscles, an increase in size (and strength) in response to use.
10. The number of occurrences per unit of time (for example, the number of activity sessions per week).

Down:
1. Length of time (for example, the time spent in each activity session).
3. Practicing an activity regularly, which leads to conditioning.
4. The capacity of the joints to move through a full range of motion; the ability to bend and recover without injury.
5. The degree of exertion while exercising (for example, the amount of weight lifted or the speed of running).
8. Becoming smaller; with regard to muscles, a decrease in size (and strength) because of disuse, undernutrition, or wasting diseases.

Match the key terms with their definitions.

11. _____ aerobic physical activity

12. _____ cardiorespiratory endurance

13. _____ heat stroke

14. _____ hyponatremia

15. _____ moderate-intensity physical activity

16. _____ muscle endurance

17. _____ muscle strength

18. _____ physical activity

19. _____ progressive overload principle

20. _____ vigorous-intensity physical activity

a. bodily movement produced by muscle contractions that substantially increase energy expenditure

b. activity in which the body's large muscles move in a rhythmic manner for a sustained period of time

c. physical activity that requires some increase in breathing and/or heart rate and expends 3.5 to 7 kcalories per minute

d. physical activity that requires a large increase in breathing and/or heart rate and expends more than 7 kcalories per minute

e. the ability of muscles to work against resistance

f. the ability of a muscle to contract repeatedly without becoming exhausted

g. the ability to perform large-muscle, dynamic exercise of moderate to high intensity for prolonged periods

h. a dangerous accumulation of body heat with accompanying loss of body fluid

i. the training principle that a body system, in order to improve, must be worked at frequencies, durations, or intensities that gradually increase physical demands

j. a decreased concentration of sodium in the blood

---

21. _____ carbohydrate loading

22. _____ cardiac output

23. _____ cardiorespiratory conditioning

24. _____ creatine phosphate

25. _____ enhanced water

26. _____ glucose polymers

27. _____ muscle power

28. _____ resistance training

29. _____ sports anemia

30. _____ VO$_2$max

a. the maximum rate of oxygen consumption by an individual at sea level

b. improvements in heart and lung function and increased blood volume, brought about by aerobic training

c. the volume of blood discharged by the heart each minute; determined by multiplying the stroke volume by the heart rate

d. the product of force generation (strength) and movement velocity (speed); the speed at which a given amount of exertion is completed

e. the use of free weights or weight machines to provide resistance for developing muscle strength, power, and endurance; also called weight training

f. a high-energy compound in muscle cells that acts as a reservoir of energy that can maintain a steady supply of ATP; provides the energy for short bursts of activity

g. a regimen of moderate exercise followed by the consumption of a high-carbohydrate diet that enables muscles to store glycogen beyond their normal capacities

h. a transient condition of low hemoglobin in the blood, associated with the early stages of sports training or other strenuous activity

i. compounds that supply glucose, not as single molecules, but linked in chains somewhat like starch

j. water that is fortified with ingredients such as vitamins, minerals, protein, oxygen, or herbs

Sample Test Questions

Select the best answer for each question.

1. The ability to meet routine physical demands with enough reserve energy to rise to a physical challenge is:
   a. physical activity.
   b. exercise.
   c. cardiorespiratory endurance.
   d. fitness.

172

2. The distinction between physical activity and exercise is:
   a. only exercise involves bodily movements and enhanced energy expenditure.
   b. physical activity benefits health more than exercise.
   c. exercise is considered more planned and structured than physical activity.
   d. exercise promotes fitness more than physical activity.

3. Lack of exercise can lead to development of:
   a. cardiovascular disease.
   b. obesity.
   c. diabetes.
   d. accelerated bone losses.
   e. All of the above

4. Benefits of fitness include:
   a. restful sleep.
   b. optimal bone density.
   c. resistance to infectious diseases such as colds.
   d. strong lung function.
   e. All of the above

5. The components of fitness include:
   a. flexibility.
   b. strength.
   c. muscle endurance.
   d. cardiorespiratory endurance.
   e. All of the above

6. Muscle response to disuse or undernutrition is called:
   a. hypertrophy.
   b. atrophy.
   c. slow-twitch fibers.
   d. fast-twitch fibers.

7. Which of the following statements is true about the progressive overload principle?
   a. It refers to practicing an activity regularly.
   b. It is the ability of the muscles to work against resistance.
   c. It refers to the idea that training must involve a gradual increase in physical demands.
   d. It focuses on the cardiorespiratory component of fitness.

8. If a person increases the length of time spent performing an activity, the progressive overload principle is being applied in what way?
   a. Duration
   b. Frequency
   c. Intensity
   d. Training

9. A person who walks at a speed of 4 miles per hour is engaging in:
   a. minimal exercise.
   b. moderate exercise.
   c. vigorous training.
   d. sedentary activity.

10. The maximum rate of oxygen consumption is:
    a. aerobic.
    b. anaerobic.
    c. the VO_2 max.
    d. cardiac output.

11. Lactate is a product of _____ metabolism.
    a. aerobic
    b. anaerobic
    c. mineral
    d. a and b
    e. a and c

12. Which of these is a high-energy compound in muscle cells that provides energy for short bursts of activity?
    a. Creatine phosphate
    b. Carbohydrate
    c. Glycogen
    d. Chromium picolinate

13. Factors that influence glycogen use during physical activity include:
    a. amount of carbohydrate in the diet.
    b. intensity and duration of the activity.
    c. degree of training to perform the activity.
    d. All of the above
    e. a and b

14. During low- or moderate-intensity activity of long duration, muscle cells use predominantly _____ as fuel.
    a. glycogen
    b. fat
    c. protein
    d. water
    e. None of the above

15. Which of the following statements is true about fat use for fuel?
    a. Fat can be used for fuel by muscles if the work is aerobic.
    b. Fat is preferred for fuel by athletes.
    c. Endurance athletes are encouraged to consume 40% of their energy from fat.
    d. Athletes on 30% fat diets experience fatigue.

16. Which of the following statements is true about fat use for fuel?
    a. Sustained, moderate activity uses body fat stores as its major fuel.
    b. As intensity of an activity increases, body fat contributes more fuel.
    c. People who are untrained will draw on fat more for fuel than those who are trained.
    d. People can burn fat from specific body parts.

17. Regarding protein and physical activity,
    a. the recommended protein intake for athletes is much higher than for non-athletes.
    b. protein is a major fuel for physical activity.
    c. synthesis of body proteins is accelerated during activity.
    d. athletes retain more protein in their muscles than nonathletes.

18. Athletes can safely add muscle tissue by:
    a. tripling their protein intake.
    b. taking hormones duplicating those of puberty.
    c. putting a demand on muscles, making them work harder.
    d. depending on protein for muscle fuel and cutting down on carbohydrates.

19. Which factor modifies the body's use of protein?
    a. Amount of carbohydrate in the diet
    b. Exercise intensity and duration
    c. The degree of training
    d. a and b
    e. a, b, and c

20. Which statement is true about vitamin/mineral supplements for athletes?
    a. All athletes should take them to improve performance.
    b. They should take supplements immediately prior to competition to enhance performance.
    c. A single daily multi-vitamin-mineral supplement that provides at least 10x the DRI is desirable.
    d. Consuming a well-balanced diet is preferable to taking supplements.

21. What element is important in the transport of oxygen in blood and muscle tissue and in energy transformation reactions?
    a. Vitamin C
    b. Zinc
    c. Iron
    d. Calcium
    e. Thiamin

22. An above-normal body temperature is
    a. hyperthermia.
    b. heat stroke.
    c. hypothermia.
    d. sports anemia

23. The first symptom of dehydration is:
    a. collapse.
    b. hunger.
    c. fatigue.
    d. chills.

24. Alcohol is a diuretic and therefore it induces:
    a. energy release.
    b. fluid losses.
    c. improved performance.
    d. iron retention.

25. The best choice for a noncompetitive exerciser who needs to rehydrate is:
    a. concentrated juice.
    b. cool water.
    c. salt tablets.
    d. sweat replacers.
    e. a or b

26. What type of athlete is most prone to iron deficiency?
    a. Male weight lifter
    b. Male swimmer
    c. Female endurance athlete
    d. Female sprinter

27. A transient condition of low hemoglobin in the blood associated with early stages of strenuous athletic training is:
    a. sports anemia.
    b. menopause.
    c. stress menstruation.
    d. amenorrhea.

28. A healthy diet for athletes consists of:
    1. nutrient-dense foods.
    2. vitamin and mineral supplements.
    3. ample fluids.
    4. salt tablets.
    5. adequate food to meet energy requirements.
    6. adequate amounts of vitamins and minerals.
    7. protein powders.

    a. 1, 2, 4, 7
    b. 1, 3, 4, 5
    c. 1, 3, 5, 6
    d. 2, 3, 4, 7
    e. 2, 4, 5, 6

29. Alcohol hinders athletic activity by:
    a. acting as a diuretic.
    b. stimulating the central nervous system.
    c. altering perceptions.
    d. a and b
    e. a and c

30. The recommended pregame meal includes:
    a. a vitamin/mineral supplement.
    b. plenty of fluids.
    c. light, easily digestible foods.
    d. b and c
    e. a, b, and c

Short Answer Questions

1. The components of fitness are:

   a.   c.

   b.   d.

2. Based on its oxygen requirements, physical activity may be classified as:

   a.   b.

3. Cardiovascular conditioning is characterized by:

   a.

   b.

   c.

   d.

   e.

   f.

4. The fuel mixture used during activity depends on:

   a.   c.

   b.

5. During endurance training, muscle cells adapt to use more _____ and less _____.

6. Active people, especially women, need to take care to consume enough _____.

7. These conditions lend themselves to hyponatremia:

   a.

   b.

8. Two poor beverage choices for athletes are:

   a.   b.

9. A healthful diet for athletes includes:

   a.   c.

   b.

Problem Solving

1. Lacey, a 38-year-old woman, plays tennis with her boyfriend for an hour on Wednesday evenings, and walks her dog for about 15 minutes each morning. How much additional activity, and what kinds of activities, should she engage in each week if she wants to meet the minimum ACSM physical fitness recommendations?

2. Jules is a 138-pound runner who regularly competes in marathons. When he is in training, what is his RDA for protein in grams per day? What is his protein requirement based on the alternative recommendation given in your text?

3. Suppose a male athlete requires 3500 kcal/day while he is in training. How many grams per day of each of the energy nutrients would a healthful diet for this athlete provide?

৬ Chapter 14 Answer Key ৶

Summing Up

1. long
2. cardiorespiratory endurance
3. adapt
4. intensity
5. glucose
6. fat
7. glycogen

8. fat
9. protein
10. supplements
11. supplements
12. iron
13. water
14. carbohydrate

15. 3
16. hyponatremia
17. training
18. nutrient-dense
19. energy
20. health
21. pregame

Chapter Study Questions

1. Fitness: the characteristics that enable the body to perform physical activity; the ability to meet routine physical demands. Benefits: more restful sleep, improved nutritional health, reduced fatness and increased lean body tissue, greater bone density, improved resistance to infectious diseases, reduced risk of some cancers, improved circulation and lung function, reduced risk of cardiovascular disease, reduced risk of type 2 diabetes, reduced risk of gallbladder disease, reduced incidence and severity of anxiety and depression, improved self-image and self-confidence, long life, and improved quality of life.

2. The training principle that a body system, in order to improve, must be worked at frequencies, durations, or intensities that gradually increase physical demands.

3. The ability to perform large-muscle, dynamic exercise of moderate-to-high intensity for prolonged periods. Benefits include support of ongoing action of the heart and lungs through increased cardiac output and oxygen delivery; increased blood volume per heartbeat (stroke volume); slower resting pulse; increased breathing efficiency; improved circulation; and reduced blood pressure.

4. Aerobic means "requiring oxygen." Thus, aerobic exercises are those that rely mostly on the oxygen-requiring metabolic pathways because the intensity is moderate enough that there is an adequate supply of oxygen for these pathways (swimming, cross-country skiing, rowing, fast walking, jogging, fast bicycling, soccer, hockey, basketball, water polo, lacrosse and rugby). Anaerobic means "not requiring oxygen," and anaerobic pathways generate energy more quickly (but less efficiently) than aerobic pathways. In terms of exercise, anaerobic refers to high-intensity activities during which the body relies mostly on anaerobic metabolic pathways to supply quick energy to meet the high demands (jump of basketball player, weight lifting, sprinting).

5. The mixture of fuels the muscles use during physical activity depends on diet, the intensity and duration of the activity, and training. During intense activity, the fuel mix is mostly glucose, whereas during less intense, moderate activity, fat makes a greater contribution. This is because oxygen is required to metabolize fat but not glucose, and thus the amount of available oxygen—which depends on the intensity of the activity and the cardiorespiratory fitness of the individual—helps to determine the proportion of energy supplied by fat. With endurance training, muscle cells adapt to store more glycogen and to rely less on glucose and more on fat for energy.

6. The body's use of glucose during physical activity depends partially on how much glycogen is in storage, and this depends partly on the amount of carbohydrate eaten. Intensity of exercise influences the body's use of glucose—high-intensity activities require more glycogen. Degree of training to perform the activity is a factor because the level of oxygen in the muscle influences the body's use of glucose. During oxygen debt, glucose is metabolized rapidly and pyruvate molecules accumulate in the muscle tissue. Duration of activity affects use of glucose during exercise—within the first 20 minutes of exercise, the body primarily uses glucose.

7. Duration of activity—when a moderate activity progresses past 20 minutes, the body uses more of its stored body fat for energy; intensity of activity—as the intensity increases, fat makes less and less of a contribution to the mixture of fuel used; degree of training—a well-trained body develops the adaptations that permit the body to draw heavily on fat for fuel.

8. Diet—people who consume diets rich in carbohydrate use less protein; intensity and duration of activity—activities more intense and long in duration will use more protein for fuel; degree of training—athletes use more protein as fuel than the unconditioned person.

9. Female athletes engaged in endurance activities are particularly likely to develop iron-deficiency anemia because of the combination of iron losses through menstruation, high demands of muscles for iron (used within mitochondria and myoglobin), and typically low intakes of iron-rich foods (especially among vegetarians). Iron-deficiency anemia is a condition that dramatically impairs physical performance. The athlete with this condition will tire easily because of impaired hemoglobin synthesis, which reduces oxygen carrying capacity of the blood. Sports anemia is a transient condition of low hemoglobin in the blood, associated with the early stage of sports training or other strenuous activity. It is an adaptive, temporary response to endurance training. Iron-deficiency anemia requires iron supplementation, whereas sports anemia does not respond to such supplementation.

10. Hydration allows the body to dissipate the heat generated by active muscles (through evaporation of sweat) and maintain proper intracellular and blood volumes. If the body loses too much water, its chemistry becomes compromised and dehydration may result. Dehydration initially causes fatigue, and can result in collapse or heat stroke in hot, humid weather. Recommendations are to drink 2-3 cups of fluid 2-3 hours prior to activity, 1-2 cups 15 minutes prior to activity, ½ to 1 cup every 15 minutes during activity, and 2 cups per pound of body weight lost after activity.

11. A nutrient-dense diet composed mostly of unprocessed foods that meets nutrient, fluid, and energy requirements. Recommended macronutrient composition: 60-70% of kcal from carbohydrate, 20-35% of kcal from fat, and 10-20% of kcal from protein. Athletes participating in intensive training should consume 6-10 g of carbohydrate per kg body weight each day.

Key Terms Practice

1. duration
2. hypothermia
3. training
4. flexibility
5. intensity
6. hyperthermia
7. conditioning
8. atrophy
9. hypertrophy
10. frequency
11. b
12. g
13. h
14. j
15. c
16. f
17. e
18. a
19. i
20. d
21. g
22. c
23. b
24. f
25. j
26. i
27. d
28. e
29. h
30. a

Sample Test Questions

1. d (p. 437)
2. c (p. 438)
3. e (pp. 438-439)
4. e (p. 438)
5. e (p. 440)
6. b (p. 441)
7. c (pp. 440-441)
8. a (p. 441)
9. b (p. 440)
10. c (p. 442)
11. b (p. 447)
12. a (p. 444)
13. d (pp. 446, 448)
14. b (p. 449)
15. a (p. 449)
16. a (p. 449)
17. d (p. 450)
18. c (p. 450)
19. e (p. 450)
20. d (pp. 451-452)
21. c (p. 452)
22. a (p. 453)
23. c (p. 453)
24. b (p. 457)
25. b (p. 454)
26. c (p. 452)
27. a (p. 453)
28. c (pp. 457-458)
29. e (p. 457)
30. d (p. 459)

Short Answer Questions

1. flexibility, muscle strength, muscle endurance, cardiorespiratory endurance

2. aerobic, anaerobic

3. increased cardiac output and oxygen delivery; increased stroke volume (blood volume per heartbeat); slowed resting pulse; increased breathing efficiency; improved circulation; reduced blood pressure

4. diet, intensity and duration of activity, training

5. fat, carbohydrate *or* glycogen

6. iron

7. excessive water intake, long endurance events with excessive loss of body fluids

8. caffeinated beverages, alcohol

9. ample fluids, variety of nutrient dense foods, foods in amounts to meet nutrient needs

Problem Solving

1. Lacey needs to increase the duration of her moderate-intensity activity to 30 minutes per day on at least 5 days of the week; she could do this by walking her dog (at a pace of 3-4 miles per hour) for an additional 15 minutes on at least 4 days of the week other than Wednesday. She also needs to add resistance activities: 2-4 sets of 9-12 repetitions for each major muscle group on 2-3 nonconsecutive days each week. Lacey should stretch after she exercises or works out, completing 2-4 stretches lasting 15-30 seconds for each muscle group.

2. RDA for protein = 0.8 g/kg/day × (138 ÷ 2.2) kg = 50 g/day
   Alternative protein level for endurance athletes = 1.2-1.4 g/kg/day × (138 ÷ 2.2) kg = 75-88 g/day

3. Carbohydrate: 60-70% × 3500 kcal = 2100-2450 kcal ÷ 4 kcal/g = 525-613 g
   Fat: 20-35% × 3500 kcal = 700-1225 kcal ÷ 9 kcal/g = 78-136 g
   Protein: 10-20% × 3500 kcal = 350-700 kcal ÷ 4 kcal/g = 88-175 g

❧ Chapter 15 – Life Cycle Nutrition: ❧
Pregnancy and Lactation

Chapter Outline

I. Nutrition Prior to Pregnancy
II. Growth and Development during Pregnancy
   A. Placental Development
   B. Fetal Growth and Development
      1. The Zygote
      2. The Embryo
      3. The Fetus
   C. Critical Periods
      1. Neural Tube Defects
      2. Folate Supplementation
      3. Chronic Diseases
      4. Fetal Programming
III. Maternal Weight
   A. Weight Prior to Conception
      1. Underweight
      2. Overweight and Obesity
   B. Weight Gain during Pregnancy
      1. Recommended Weight Gains
      2. Weight-Gain Patterns
      3. Components of Weight Gain
      4. Weight Loss after Pregnancy
   C. Exercise during Pregnancy
IV. Nutrition during Pregnancy
   A. Energy and Nutrient Needs during Pregnancy
      1. Energy
      2. Carbohydrate
      3. Protein
      4. Essential Fatty Acids
      5. Nutrients for Blood Production and Cell Growth
      6. Nutrients for Bone Development
      7. Other Nutrients
      8. Nutrient Supplements
   B. Vegetarian Diets during Pregnancy and Lactation
   C. Common Nutrition-Related Concerns of Pregnancy
      1. Nausea and Vomiting
      2. Constipation and Hemorrhoids
      3. Heartburn
      4. Food Cravings and Aversions
      5. Nonfood Cravings
V. High-Risk Pregnancies
   A. The Infant's Birthweight
   B. Malnutrition and Pregnancy
      1. Malnutrition and Fertility
      2. Malnutrition and Early Pregnancy
      3. Malnutrition and Fetal Development
   C. Food Assistance Programs

   D. Maternal Health
      1. Preexisting Diabetes
      2. Gestational Diabetes
      3. Chronic Hypertension
      4. Gestational Hypertension
      5. Preeclampsia
   E. The Mother's Age
      1. Pregnancy in Adolescents
      2. Pregnancy in Older Women
   F. Practices Incompatible with Pregnancy
      1. Alcohol
      2. Medicinal Drugs
      3. Herbal Supplements
      4. Illicit Drugs
      5. Smoking and Chewing Tobacco
      6. Environmental Contaminants
      7. Foodborne Illness
      8. Vitamin-Mineral Megadoses
      9. Caffeine
      10. Restrictive Dieting
      11. Sugar Substitutes
VI. Nutrition during Lactation
   A. Lactation: A Physiological Process
   B. Breastfeeding: A Learned Behavior
   C. Maternal Energy and Nutrient Needs during Lactation
      1. Energy Intake and Exercise
      2. Energy Nutrients
      3. Vitamins and Minerals
      4. Water
      5. Nutrient Supplements
      6. Food Assistance Programs
      7. Particular Foods
   D. Maternal Health
      1. HIV Infection and AIDS
      2. Diabetes
      3. Postpartum Amenorrhea
      4. Breast Health
   E. Practices Incompatible with Lactation
      1. Alcohol
      2. Medicinal Drugs
      3. Illicit Drugs
      4. Smoking
      5. Environmental Contaminants
      6. Caffeine
VII. Fetal Alcohol Syndrome
   A. Drinking during Pregnancy
   B. How Much Is Too Much?
   C. When Is the Damage Done?

180

Summing Up

Prior to pregnancy, the health and behaviors of both 1._____ and women can influence 2._____ and fetal development. In preparation, they can achieve and maintain a healthy body weight, choose an 3._____ and balanced diet, be physically active, receive regular 4._____ care, manage chronic conditions, and avoid 5._____ influences.

Maternal nutrition before and during pregnancy affects both the mother's 6._____ and the infant's growth. As the infant develops through its three stages—the 7._____, embryo, and fetus—its organs and tissues grow, each on its own schedule. Times of intense development are 8._____ _____ that depend on nutrients to proceed smoothly. Without folate, for example, the 9._____ _____ fails to develop completely during the first month of pregnancy, prompting recommendations that all women of childbearing age take 10._____ daily.

A healthy pregnancy depends on a sufficient 11._____ gain. Women who begin their pregnancies at a healthy weight need to gain about 12._____ pounds, which covers the growth and development of the placenta, 13._____, blood, breasts, and infant. By remaining 14._____ throughout pregnancy, a woman can develop the 15._____ she needs to carry the extra weight and maintain habits that will help her lose weight after the birth.

Energy and nutrient needs are 16._____ during pregnancy. A balanced diet that includes an extra serving from each of the five 17._____ _____ can usually meet these needs, with the possible exception of 18._____ and folate (supplements are recommended). The nausea, 19._____, and heartburn that sometimes accompany pregnancy can usually be alleviated with a few simple strategies. Food cravings do not typically reflect 20._____ needs.

21._____-_____ pregnancies, especially for teenagers, threaten the life and health of both mother and infant. Proper nutrition and abstinence from 22._____, 23._____, and other drugs improve the outcome. In addition, prenatal care includes monitoring pregnant women for gestational 24._____, gestational hypertension, and 25._____.

The lactating woman needs extra 26._____ and enough 27._____ and nutrients to produce about 25 ounces of milk a day. Breastfeeding is contraindicated for those with 28._____. 29._____, other drugs, smoking, and contaminants may reduce milk 30._____ or enter breast milk and impair infant development.

Chapter Study Questions

1. List ways men and women can prepare for a healthy pregnancy.

2. Describe the placenta and its function.

3. Describe the normal events of fetal development. How does malnutrition impair fetal development?

4. Define the term *critical period*. How do adverse influences during critical periods affect later health?

5. Explain why women of childbearing age need folate in their diets. How much is recommended, and how can women ensure that these needs are met?

6. What is the recommended pattern of weight gain during pregnancy for a woman at a healthy weight? For an underweight woman? For an overweight woman? For an obese woman?

7. What does a pregnant woman need to know about exercise?

8. Which nutrients are needed in the greatest amounts during pregnancy? Why are they so important? Describe wise food choices for the pregnant woman.

9. Define low-risk and high-risk pregnancies. What is the significance of infant birthweight in terms of the child's future health?

182

10. Describe some of the special problems of the pregnant adolescent.

11. What practices should be avoided during pregnancy? Why?

12. How do nutrient needs during lactation differ from nutrient needs during pregnancy?

Key Terms Practice

To complete the crossword puzzle, identify the key term that best matches each definition.

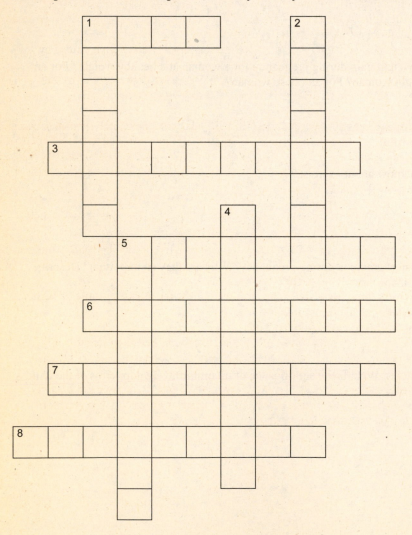

Across:

1. The general term for eating nonfood items.
3. The period from conception to birth.
5. The organ that develops inside the uterus early in pregnancy, through which the fetus receives nutrients and oxygen and returns carbon dioxide and other waste products to be excreted.
6. A hormone secreted from the anterior pituitary gland that acts on the mammary glands to promote the production of milk.
7. The union of the male sperm and the female ovum; fertilization.
8. The capacity of a woman to produce a normal ovum periodically and of a man to produce normal sperm; the ability to reproduce.

Down:
1. Prior to the thirty-eighth week of pregnancy.
2. A hormone that stimulates the mammary glands to eject milk during lactation and the uterus to contract during childbirth.
4. A severe stage of preeclampsia characterized by seizures.
5. Referring to the time between the twenty-eighth week of gestation and one month after birth.

Match the key terms with their definitions.

9. _____ anencephaly

10. _____ critical periods

11. _____ full term

12. _____ gestational diabetes

13. _____ gestational hypertension

14. _____ neural tube defect

15. _____ postpartum amenorrhea

16. _____ preeclampsia

17. _____ spina bifida

18. _____ sudden infant death syndrome

a. the normal temporary absence of menstrual periods immediately following childbirth
b. the unexpected and unexplained death of an apparently well infant; the most common cause of death of infants between the second week and the end of the first year of life
c. glucose intolerance with onset or first recognition during pregnancy
d. finite periods during development in which certain events occur that will have irreversible effects on later developmental stages; usually a period of rapid cell division
e. a condition characterized by hypertension and protein in the urine
f. between the thirty-eighth and forty-second week of pregnancy
g. high blood pressure that develops in the second half of pregnancy and resolves after childbirth, usually without affecting the outcome of the pregnancy
h. malformations of the brain, spinal cord, or both during embryonic development that often results in lifelong disability or death
i. an uncommon and always fatal type of neural tube defect; characterized by the absence of a brain
j. one of the most common types of neural tube defects; characterized by the incomplete closure of the spinal cord and its bony encasement

19. _____ cesarean section

20. _____ fetal programming

21. _____ food cravings

22. _____ food aversions

23. _____ high-risk pregnancy

24. _____ listeriosis

25. _____ low birthweight

26. _____ low-risk pregnancy

27. _____ macrosomia

28. _____ post term

a. the influence of substances during fetal growth on the development of diseases in later life
b. a pregnancy characterized by risk factors that make it likely the birth will be surrounded by problems such as premature delivery, difficult birth, restricted growth, birth defects, and early infant death
c. after the forty-second week of pregnancy
d. a surgically assisted birth involving removal of the fetus by an incision into the uterus, usually by way of the abdominal wall
e. a pregnancy characterized by factors that make it likely the birth will be normal and the infant healthy
f. strong desires to avoid particular foods
g. abnormally large body size, e.g., a birthweight at the 90th percentile or higher for gestational age for an infant
h. strong desires to eat particular foods
i. a birthweight of 5½ pounds (2500 grams) or less; indicates probable poor health in the newborn and poor nutrition status in the mother during pregnancy, before pregnancy, or both
j. an infection caused by eating food contaminated with the bacterium *Listeria monocytogenes*, which can be killed by pasteurization and cooking but can survive at refrigerated temperatures

Sample Test Questions

Select the best answer for each question.

1. The capacity of men and women to reproduce is:
   a. implantation.
   b. gestation.
   c. fertility.
   d. ferrum.

2. The union of the male sperm and female ovum is called:
   a. a zygote.
   b. conception.
   c. a blastocyst.
   d. a placenta.

3. The product of the union of the male sperm and female ovum is called:
   a. a zygote.
   b. conception.
   c. fertilization.
   d. a fetus.

4. The muscular organ within which the infant develops before birth is the:
   a. placenta.
   b. amniotic sac.
   c. vagina.
   d. uterus.

5. The structure through which the fetus's veins and arteries reach the placenta is the:
   a. umbilical cord.
   b. ovum.
   c. amniotic sac.
   d. fallopian tube.

6. In preparation for a healthy pregnancy, women can establish the following habits:
   a. maintain a healthy body weight and be physically active.
   b. consume an adequate and healthy diet, and receive regular medical care.
   c. select high levels of vitamin/mineral supplements and low-impact exercises.
   d. a and b
   e. a and c

7. Nutrients and oxygen travel to the developing fetus via:
   a. the placenta.
   b. the amniotic sac.
   c. its lungs.
   d. its intestines.

8. The growth period when a lack of nutrients is most likely to produce permanent change is the:
   a. period of rapid increase in number of cells.
   b. period of rapid increase in size of cells.
   c. teen growth spurt.
   d. third trimester of pregnancy.

9. A fetus is the:
   a. developing infant during its second through eighth week after conception.
   b. developing infant from the eighth week after conception until birth.
   c. muscular organ within which the infant develops before birth.
   d. infant from birth until its first birthday.
   e. organ from which the infant receives nourishment.

10. The critical period for neural tube development is from:
    a. 17 to 30 days gestation.
    b. 31 to 40 days gestation.
    c. 41 to 60 days gestation.
    d. 61 to 70 days gestation.

11. Neural tube defects result in the following condition(s):
    a. spina bifida.
    b. anencephaly.
    c. macrosomia.
    d. a and c
    e. a and b

185

12. A pregnant woman (compared to a non-pregnant woman) is advised to consume 1.5 times as much:
    a. food energy (kcalories).
    b. calcium.
    c. fat.
    d. carbohydrate.
    e. folate.

13. Which of the following statements is true regarding pregnancy and chronic diseases?
    a. Adverse influences at critical times are not related to chronic diseases later in life.
    b. Poor maternal diet may influence blood pressure but not immune functions.
    c. Malnutrition is not an influence on type 2 diabetes.
    d. Low birth weight and premature birth correlate with insulin resistance.

14. The influence of substances during fetal growth on the development of diseases later in life is:
    a. gestational diabetes.
    b. fetal programming.
    c. high-risk pregnancy.
    d. Down syndrome.

15. An infant born prior to the 38th week of pregnancy is:
    a. term.
    b. post term.
    c. preterm.
    d. low risk.

16. A surgically assisted birth involving an incision into the uterus is called:
    a. vaginal delivery.
    b. cesarean section.
    c. eclampsia.
    d. episiotomy.

17. Strong desires to avoid certain foods are:
    a. food cravings.
    b. food intolerances.
    c. food allergies.
    d. food aversions.

18. High-birthweight infants are called:
    a. post term.
    b. macrosomic.
    c. macroscelian.
    d. macrogametes.

19. For women who begin pregnancy at a healthy weight, physicians often recommend:
    a. weight gain of about 25 to 35 pounds.
    b. no mineral or vitamin supplements and weight gain of at least 35 pounds.
    c. vitamin C supplements and weight gain of about 20 pounds.
    d. multi-vitamin and -mineral supplements and weight gain of no more than 20 pounds.

20. Because of the dangers of obesity, an overweight pregnant woman should try to gain:
    a. 25 to 28 pounds during pregnancy.
    b. 28 to 40 pounds during pregnancy.
    c. 15 to 25 pounds during pregnancy.
    d. no weight during pregnancy.

21. A severe condition characterized by hypertension, protein in the urine, seizures, and possibly coma is:
    a. gestational diabetes.
    b. preeclampsia.
    c. eclampsia.
    d. SIDS.

22. Which of the following statements is true regarding nutrition during pregnancy?
    a. Damage done to an infant by a woman's alcohol abuse during pregnancy can be corrected after birth by proper nutrition.
    b. The RDA for vitamin D increases during pregnancy.
    c. The iron RDA during pregnancy is 27 mg/day.
    d. Calcium absorption and retention decrease during pregnancy.

23. Vegan diets during pregnancy:
    a. always result in low-birthweight babies that have statistically greater chances of contracting diseases and of dying early in life.
    b. do not require any supplementation.
    c. require iron supplementation.
    d. do not require calcium supplementation.

24. The stage of development in which the fertilized egg embeds itself in the wall of the uterus is called:
    a. the ovum.
    d. the zygote.
    b. the critical period.
    e. implantation.
    c. the placenta.

25. A pregnant woman who is constipated asks a health care provider for advice. Assuming no disease is present, what should the health care provider probably tell her to try first?
    a. Increase fluid intake
    c. Eat fewer bulky foods
    b. Use laxatives
    d. Reduce fluid intake

26. During the second trimester, a pregnant woman needs _____ kcalories above the allowance for a nonpregnant woman.
    a. 340
    c. 530
    b. 450
    d. 620

27. The protein RDA for pregnancy is _____ grams per day higher than for nonpregnant women.
    a. 2
    c. 10
    b. 6
    d. 25

28. The increased need for _____ in pregnancy is difficult to meet by diet or by existing stores; therefore supplements are recommended.
    a. vitamin C
    c. iron
    b. sodium
    d. vitamin D

29. The most common outcome of a high-risk pregnancy is:
    a. diabetes.
    c. weight appropriate for gestational age.
    b. heart disease.
    d. low birthweight.

30. Pregnant teenagers have high rates of
    a. stillbirths.
    d. All of the above
    b. preterm births.
    e. b and c
    c. low-birthweight infants.

Short Answer Questions

1. Prior to pregnancy, the health and behaviors of both men and women can influence:

    a.   b.

2. In preparation for a healthy pregnancy, men and women can:

    a.

    b.

    c.

    d.

    e.

    f.

3. Factors that increase the likelihood of a neural tube defect during pregnancy include:

   a.

   b.

   c:

   d.

   e.

4. Three stages of infant development after fertilization are:

   a.   b.

   c.

5. Two characteristics of the mother's weight that influence an infant's birthweight are:

   a.

   b.

6. Components of healthy weight gain during pregnancy include:

   a.   e.

   b.   f.

   c.   g.

   d.

7. Two nutrient supplements that are recommended for women during pregnancy are:

   a.   b.

8. Nutrition advice that is disseminated in prenatal care includes:

   a.

   b.

   c.

   d.

9. Consequences of malnutrition during pregnancy include:

   a.   d.

   b.   e.

   c.   f.

10. WIC foods are selected to supply these nutrients known to be lacking in the diets of the target population:

   a.   d.

   b.   e.

   c.

188

11. Medical disorders that can threaten the life and health of both mother and fetus include:

    a.   d.

    b.   e.

    c.

12. Complications associated with smoking during pregnancy include:

    a.   e.

    b.   f.

    c.   g.

    d.   h.

13. WIC incentives to breastfeed include:

    a.

    b.

    c.

    d.

14. Practices incompatible with lactation include:

    a.   d.

    b.   e.

    c.   f.

Problem Solving

1. What is the recommended energy intake during the 2nd and 3rd trimesters of pregnancy for a woman at a healthy weight whose non-pregnancy estimated energy expenditure is 1800 kcalories?

2. Ideally, how much weight would you expect a normal-weight woman to have gained by the 32nd week of pregnancy?

❧ Chapter 15 Answer Key ❧

Summing Up

1. men	9. neural tube	17. food groups	25. preeclampsia
2. fertility	10. folate	18. iron	26. fluid
3. adequate	11. weight	19. constipation	27. energy
4. medical	12. 30 *or* 25-35	20. physiological	28. HIV/AIDS
5. harmful	13. uterus	21. High-risk	29. Alcohol
6. health	14. active	22. smoking	30. production
7. zygote	15. strength	23. alcohol	
8. critical periods	16. high	24. diabetes	

Chapter Study Questions

1. Prior to pregnancy, the health and behaviors of both men and women can influence fertility and fetal development. In preparation, they can achieve and maintain a healthy body weight, choose an adequate and balanced diet, be physically active, receive regular medical care, manage chronic conditions, and avoid harmful influences.

2. The placenta is the organ that develops inside the uterus early in pregnancy, in which maternal and fetal blood circulate in close proximity so that materials can be exchanged between them. The baby receives nutrients and oxygen across the placenta, and the mother's blood picks up carbon dioxide and other waste products to be excreted.

3. During the 7 months of fetal development, each organ grows to maturity according to its own characteristic schedule, with greater intensity at some times than at others. Intense development and rapid cell division take place only during certain times, known as critical periods. During these times, each organ and tissue undergoing rapid development is most vulnerable to an insult such as a nutrient deficiency. If nutrients are not available during these times, that organ or tissue may develop abnormally, resulting in birth defects.

4. Critical periods are finite periods during development in which certain events may occur that will have irreversible effects on later developmental stages. In the case of the developing fetus, a critical period is a period of rapid cell division. Malnutrition during these times affects the organ systems undergoing a critical period of development, and these negative effects (e.g., birth defects) persist in later life.

5. Folate is needed for closure of the neural tube (which develops into the spinal cord), and hence can prevent neural tube defects. 0.4 mg/day is recommended; women should eat plenty of fruits, vegetables, and fortified foods or take supplements.

6. Total recommended weight gain for underweight: 28 to 40 lb.; normal-weight: 25 to 35 lb.; overweight: 15 to 25 lb.; obese: 11-20 lb. For a normal-weight woman, the appropriate pattern is to gain 3.5 lb. during the first trimester and ~1 lb./week thereafter. Underweight women should gain ~5 lb. during the first trimester and just over 1 lb./week thereafter; overweight women, ~2 lb. in the first trimester and then $^2/_3$ lb./week thereafter.

7. A woman who is active prior to pregnancy and is experiencing a normal pregnancy can continue to exercise throughout her pregnancy, but will want to choose low-impact activities and avoid sports in which she might fall or be hit by other people or objects such as racquetball. Women are advised to avoid overly strenuous activities and to abstain from exercising in hot weather, and to stay out of saunas, steam rooms, and hot whirlpools.

8. Energy nutrients are essential (a women needs extra food energy to support the growth and metabolic activities of the placenta, fetus, and her own body tissues), extra protein is needed for growth of new tissues, additional B vitamins are needed in proportion to increased food energy intake (they function as coenzymes in energy reactions), folate and B_{12} are needed for blood cells and growth, vitamin D and minerals are necessary for bone development, extra iron is needed to provide for fetal and placental needs and usually to boost pre-pregnancy low blood levels, and zinc is needed for DNA and RNA synthesis (thus for protein synthesis and cell development). Wise food choices include a balance similar to that of the USDA Food Patterns with additional

portions for each of the five food groups to meet increased nutrient needs (based on amounts recommended for the higher kcal intakes during the second and third trimesters).

9. Low-risk pregnancy: a pregnancy characterized by factors that make it likely the birth will be normal and the infant healthy; high-risk pregnancy: a pregnancy characterized by risk factors that make it likely the birth will be surrounded by problems such as premature delivery, difficult birth, restricted growth, birth defects, and early infant death. Birthweight is a reliable predictor of an infant's future health and survival.

10. A teenaged female is growing and has to meet her own nutrient needs, in addition to trying to meet the nutrient needs of a developing baby. The demands of pregnancy compete with those of her own growth, placing her and the infant at high risk for complications such as iron-deficiency anemia, prolonged labor, stillbirths, preterm births, and low infant birthweight. Adolescents typically have few financial resources and so have poor access to prenatal care.

11. Drinking alcohol, taking medicinal drugs not approved by a physician, using illicit drugs, smoking or using smokeless tobacco, ingesting foods and beverages contaminated with lead or mercury, consuming foods that pose a risk of foodborne illness, taking vitamin-mineral megadoses, drinking excessive caffeine, and restrictive dieting. Substances such as alcohol and drugs can pass to the fetus and cause irreversible harm or death. Smoking restricts the oxygen delivery to the fetus. Heavy metal exposure retards mental development, and restrictive dieting can result in a low-birth weight infant. Foods that have not been safely handled/cooked can transmit pathogens that harm the fetus.

12. In general, nutrient needs are as high or higher during lactation as during pregnancy (exceptions are iron, magnesium, and folate).

Key Terms Practice

1. A: pica;
   D: preterm
2. oxytocin
3. gestation
4. eclampsia
5. A: placenta;
   D: perinatal
6. prolactin
7. conception
8. fertility
9. i
10. d
11. f
12. c
13. g
14. h
15. a
16. e
17. j
18. b
19. d
20. a
21. h
22. f
23. b
24. j
25. i
26. e
27. g
28. c

Sample Test Questions

1. c (p. 469)
2. b (p. 470)
3. a (p. 471)
4. d (p. 470)
5. a (p. 471)
6. d (p. 470)
7. a (pp. 470, 471)
8. a (p. 472)
9. b (p. 472)
10. a (p. 472)
11. e (p. 473)
12. e (p. 474, 481)
13. d (p. 475)
14. b (p. 475)
15. c (p. 476)
16. b (p. 476)
17. d (p. 484)
18. b (p. 476)
19. a (pp. 476-477)
20. c (pp. 476-477)
21. c (p. 487)
22. c (pp. 481-482)
23. c (p. 483)
24. e (p. 471)
25. a (p. 483)
26. a (p. 480)
27. d (p. 480)
28. c (pp. 481-482)
29. d (p. 484)
30. d (p. 488)

Short Answer Questions

1. fertility, fetal development

2. achieve and maintain a healthy body weight; choose an adequate and balanced diet; be physically active; receive regular medical care; manage chronic conditions; avoid harmful influences

3. a personal or family history of a pregnancy affected by a neural tube defect, maternal diabetes, maternal use of certain antiseizure medications, mutations in folate-related enzymes, maternal obesity

4. zygote, embryo, fetus

5. her weight prior to conception, her weight gain during pregnancy.

6. placenta, uterus, blood, breasts, increased blood supply and fluid volume, infant, maternal fat stores

7. iron, folate

8. eat well-balanced meals; gain enough weight to support fetal growth; take prenatal supplements as prescribed; stop drinking alcohol

9. fetal growth restriction, congenital malformations (birth defects), spontaneous abortion, stillbirth, preterm birth, low infant birthweight

10. protein, calcium, iron, vitamin A, vitamin C

11. preexisting diabetes, gestational diabetes, chronic hypertension, gestational hypertension, preeclampsia

12. fetal growth restriction, preterm birth, low birthweight, premature separation of the placenta, miscarriage, stillbirth, sudden infant death syndrome (SIDS), congenital malformations

13. higher priority in certification into WIC, longer eligibility to participate in WIC, more foods and larger quantities, breast pumps and other support materials

14. alcohol use, use of some medicinal drugs, use of illicit drugs, smoking, exposure to environmental contaminants, caffeine use

Problem Solving

1. 1800 + 340 kcalories per day during 2nd trimester = 2140 kcalories
   1800 + 450 kcalories per day during 3rd trimester = 2250 kcalories

2. 3.5 lb./1st 3 mo (13 wk) + 19 wk × 1 lb./week = 3.5 + 19 = 22.5 lb.

◎ Chapter 16 – Life Cycle Nutrition: ◎ Infancy, Childhood, and Adolescence

Chapter Outline

I. Nutrition during Infancy
  A. Energy and Nutrient Needs
    1. Energy Intake and Activity
    2. Energy Nutrients
    3. Vitamins and Minerals
    4. Water
  B. Breast Milk
    1. Frequency and Duration of Breastfeeding
    2. Energy Nutrients
    3. Vitamins
    4. Minerals
    5. Supplements
    6. Immunological Protection
    7. Allergy and Disease Protection
    8. Other Potential Benefits
    9. Breast Milk Banks
  C. Infant Formula
    1. Infant Formula Composition
    2. Risks of Formula Feeding
    3. Infant Formula Standards
    4. Special Formulas
    5. Inappropriate Formulas
    6. Nursing Bottle Tooth Decay
  D. Special Needs of Preterm Infants
  E. Introducing Cow's Milk
  F. Introducing Solid Foods
    1. When to Begin
    2. Food Allergies
    3. Choice of Infant Foods
    4. Foods to Provide Iron
    5. Foods to Provide Vitamin C
    6. Foods to Omit
    7. Vegetarian Diets during Infancy
    8. Foods at 1 Year
  G. Mealtimes with Toddlers
II. Nutrition during Childhood
  A. Energy and Nutrient Needs
    1. Energy Intake and Activity
    2. Carbohydrate and Fiber
    3. Fat and Fatty Acids
    4. Protein
    5. Vitamins and Minerals
    6. Supplements
    7. Planning Children's Meals
  B. Hunger and Malnutrition in Children
    1. Hunger and Behavior
    2. Iron Deficiency and Behavior

    3. Other Nutrient Deficiencies and Behavior
  C. The Malnutrition-Lead Connection
  D. Hyperactivity and "Hyper" Behavior
    1. Hyperactivity
    2. Misbehaving
  E. Food Allergy and Intolerance
    1. Detecting Food Allergy
    2. Anaphylactic Shock
    3. Food Labeling
    4. Food Intolerances
  F. Childhood Obesity
    1. Genetic and Environmental Factors
    2. Growth
    3. Physical Health
    4. Psychological Development
    5. Prevention and Treatment of Obesity
    6. Diet
    7. Physical Activity
    8. Psychological Support
    9. Behavioral Changes
    10. Drugs
    11. Surgery
  G. Mealtimes at Home
    1. Honoring Children's Preferences
    2. Learning through Participation
    3. Avoiding Power Struggles
    4. Choking Prevention
    5. Playing First
    6. Snacking
    7. Preventing Dental Caries
    8. Serving as Role Models
  H. Nutrition at School
    1. Meals at School
    2. Competing Influences at School
III. Nutrition during Adolescence
  A. Growth and Development
  B. Energy and Nutrient Needs
    1. Energy Intake and Activity
    2. Vitamins
    3. Iron
    4. Calcium
  C. Food Choices and Health Habits
    1. Snacks
    2. Beverages
    3. Eating Away from Home
    4. Peer Influence

IV. Childhood Obesity and the Early Development
of Chronic Diseases
  A. Early Development of Type 2 Diabetes
  B. Early Development of Heart Disease
    1. Atherosclerosis
    2. Blood Cholesterol
    3. Blood Pressure
  C. Physical Activity
  D. Dietary Recommendations for Children
    1. Moderation, Not Deprivation
    2. Diet First, Drugs Later
  E. Smoking

Summing Up

The primary food for infants during the first 12 months is either 1._____ _____ or iron-fortified 2._____. In addition to nutrients, breast milk also offers 3._____ protection. At about 4 to 6 months of age, infants should gradually begin eating 4._____ foods. By 1 year, they are drinking from a cup and eating many of the 5._____ foods as the rest of the family.

Children's appetites and nutrient needs reflect their stage of 6._____. Those who are chronically hungry and malnourished suffer growth 7._____; when hunger is temporary and nutrient deficiencies are mild, the problems are usually more 8._____—such as poor academic performance. Iron deficiency is widespread and has many physical and 9._____ consequences. "Hyper" behavior is not caused by poor nutrition; misbehavior may be due to lack of 10._____, too little physical activity, or too much 11._____, among other factors. Childhood 12._____ has become a major health problem. Adults at home and at school need to provide children with 13._____-_____ foods and teach them how to make healthful diet and 14._____ choices.

Nutrient needs rise dramatically as children enter the 15._____ growth phase of adolescence. Teenagers' busy lifestyles add to the challenge of meeting their 16._____ needs, especially for iron and 17._____.

Chapter Study Questions

1. Describe some of the nutrient and immunological attributes of breast milk.

2. What are the appropriate uses of formula feeding? What criteria would you use in selecting an infant formula?

3. Why are solid foods not recommended for an infant during the first few months of life? When is an infant ready to start eating solid food?

194

4. Identify foods that are inappropriate for infants and explain why they are inappropriate.

5. What micronutrient deficiencies are most common in U.S. children? What strategies can help prevent them?

6. Describe the relationship between nutrition and behavior. How does television influence nutrition?

7. Describe a true food allergy. Which foods most often cause allergic reactions? How do food allergies influence nutrition status?

8. Describe the problems associated with childhood obesity and the strategies for prevention and treatment.

9. List strategies for introducing nutritious foods to children.

10. What impact do school meal programs have on the nutrition status of children?

11. Describe changes in nutrient needs from childhood to adolescence. Why is a teenaged girl more likely to develop an iron deficiency than is a boy?

12. How do adolescents' eating habits influence their nutrient intakes?

Key Terms Practice

To complete the crossword puzzle, identify the key term that best matches each definition.

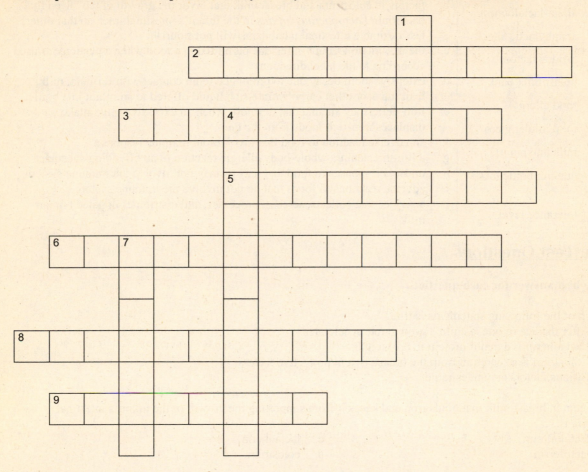

Across:

2. A protein in breast milk that binds iron and keeps it from supporting the growth of the infant's intestinal bacteria.
3. The period from the beginning of puberty until maturity.
5. A milklike secretion from the breast, present during the first few days after delivery before milk appears; rich in protective factors.
6. Inattentive and impulsive behavior that is more frequent and severe than is typical of others a similar age.
8. With respect to nutrition, key people who control other people's access to foods and thereby exert profound impacts on their nutrition.
9. An often fatal foodborne illness caused by the ingestion of foods containing a toxin produced by bacteria that grow without oxygen.

Down:

1. To gradually replace breast milk with infant formula or other foods appropriate to an infant's diet.
4. A protein in breast milk that attacks diarrhea-causing viruses.
7. The period in life in which a person becomes physically capable of reproduction.

Match the key terms with their definitions.

10. _____ adverse reactions

11. _____ alpha-lactalbumin

12. _____ anaphylactic shock

13. _____ bifidus factors

14. _____ breast milk bank

15. _____ food allergy

16. _____ food intolerances

17. _____ milk anemia

18. _____ nursing bottle tooth decay

19. _____ tolerance level

a. a major protein in human breast milk

b. factors in colostrum and breast milk that favor the growth of the "friendly" bacterium *Lactobacillus bifidus* in the infant's intestinal tract, so that other, less desirable intestinal inhabitants will not flourish

c. the maximum amount of residue permitted in a food when a pesticide is used according to the label directions

d. extensive tooth decay due to prolonged tooth contact with formula, milk, fruit juice, or other carbohydrate-rich liquid offered to an infant in a bottle

e. iron-deficiency anemia that develops when an excessive milk intake displaces iron-rich foods from the diet

f. an adverse reaction to food that involves an immune response

g. a life-threatening, whole-body allergic reaction to an offending substance

h. unusual responses to food that may or may not involve the immune system

i. adverse reactions to foods that do not involve the immune system

j. a service that collects, screens, processes, and distributes donated human milk

Sample Test Questions

Select the best answer for each question.

1. Which of the following statements is true?
   a. After the age of one, a child's growth rate accelerates.
   b. Lactadherin is a major protein in breast milk.
   c. Colostrum is a secretion from the breast, rich in protective factors.
   d. Bifidus factors are undesirable.

2. A protein in breast milk that binds iron and keeps it from supporting the growth of the infant's intestinal bacteria is:
   a. lactalbumin.
   b. lactoferrin.
   c. lactadherin.
   d. colostrum.

3. The American Academy of Pediatrics recommends that:
   a. infants exclusively receive breast milk for the first 6 months.
   b. infants receive breast milk and complementary foods for 3 to 6 months.
   c. infants receive breast milk or formula for the first 12 months.
   d. infants exclusively receive breast milk for the first 3 years.

4. Since breast milk contains relatively low levels of iron,
   a. iron supplementation may be suggested.
   b. formula feeding is preferred.
   c. iron has a low bioavailability.
   d. feeding liver to the infant is suggested.

5. Benefits of breastfeeding include:
   a. immunological protection, including colostrum, which contains antibodies.
   b. bifidus factors that favor the growth of friendly bacteria in the infant's digestive tract.
   c. lactoferrin and lactadherin that protect against infant diarrhea.
   d. protection against allergy development.
   e. All of the above

6. At what age can a normal infant begin eating solid foods?
   a. 3-5 weeks
   b. 26-32 weeks
   c. 4-6 months
   d. 9-12 months

7. What should be the first food introduced to the infant?
   a. Yogurt
   b. Egg white
   c. Rice cereal
   d. Finely chopped meat

8. The main purpose of introducing solid food is:
   a. to help the infant sleep through the night.
   b. to provide nutrients that are no longer supplied adequately by breast milk alone.
   c. to increase body weight.
   d. to improve mental capacity.

9. Which of the following changes in body structure usually takes place between the ages of 1 and 2 years?
   a. Weight doubles
   b. Weight triples
   c. Length of body doubles
   d. Length of long bones increases

10. Approximately how many kcalories per day does an average 1-year old need to obtain?
    a. 500
    b. 800
    c. 1300
    d. 2400

11. Which of the following provides the most important information about a child's health?
    a. Growth chart
    b. Blood lipid profile
    c. Long-bone size and density
    d. Onset of walking and talking

12. A two year old requiring 1000 kcal/day needs _____ cups from the milk group daily.
    a. one
    b. one-half
    c. two
    d. three

13. A large amount of concentrated sweets in a child's diet is most likely to lead to:
    a. apathy.
    b. obesity.
    c. hyperactivity.
    d. growth inhibition.

14. An adverse reaction to foods that does not involve an immune response is:
    a. a food intolerance.
    b. a food allergy.
    c. an antigen.
    d. anaphylactic shock.

15. Inattentive and impulsive behavior that is more frequent and severe than is typical of others of a similar age is:
    a. hypoallergenic.
    b. hyperactivity.
    c. obsessive-compulsive disorder.
    d. adversive behavior.

16. How much more total energy does a normal 10 year old need compared with a normal 1 year old?
    a. 25%
    b. 50%
    c. 150%
    d. 200%

17. Which of the following two conditions are associated with frequent television viewing?
    a. Obesity and inactivity
    b. Drug abuse and teenage pregnancy
    c. Anorexia and nutrient deficiencies
    d. Hyperactivity and lower body weight

18. Compared with adolescent boys in terms of height, weight, and body composition, adolescent girls:
    a. start growing later.
    b. gain more fat mass.
    c. have more lean body mass.
    d. have more energy.

19. The School Lunch Program is intended to provide at least _____ of children's RDA for certain nutrients.
    a. one fourth
    b. one third
    c. one hundred percent
    d. No requirement stipulated.

198

20. Which of the following statements is true regarding obesity?
    a. The number of overweight children has remained steady over the past four decades.
    b. Parental obesity is not correlated with childhood obesity.
    c. Diet and physical activity are unrelated to childhood obesity.
    d. Soft drink intake and fast food consumption play roles in childhood weight gains.

21. Key people who control other people's access to foods are called:
    a. gatekeepers.
    b. food monitors.
    c. chiefs.
    d. food directors.

22. One nutrient that often comes up short in teenagers' diets is:
    a. protein.
    b. sodium.
    c. thiamin.
    d. iron.
    e. riboflavin.

23. A negative influence on nutrition in schools is:
    a. reimbursable foods.
    b. the School Breakfast Program.
    c. foods from vending machines.
    d. All of the above

24. Adolescents who drink more soft drinks and less milk
    a. have high intakes of iron.
    b. have high intakes of calcium.
    c. have high intakes of fat.
    d. have low energy intakes.
    e. are more likely to be overweight.

25. The single most effective way to teach nutrition to children is by:
    a. example.
    b. punishment.
    c. singling out only hazardous nutrition practices for attention.
    d. explaining the importance of eating new foods as a prerequisite for dessert.

26. What can parents do to help their children consume a balanced diet?
    a. Allow eating only at mealtimes and forbid all snacking.
    b. Make a variety of nutritious foods available.
    c. Insist on keeping close track of everything they eat.
    d. Parents really can't do anything to influence their diets.

27. A teenager's kcalorie intake from snacks typically represents at least _____ percent of total daily intake.
    a. five
    b. fifteen
    c. twenty-five
    d. forty
    e. fifty

28. Low calcium intake during adolescence can:
    a. result in anemia.
    b. prevent growth spurts.
    c. compromise the development of peak bone mass.
    d. reduce white blood cell count.

29. _____ increases susceptibility to lead poisoning, and these two conditions have similar symptoms.
    a. Iron toxicity
    b. Iron deficiency
    c. Vitamin C deficiency
    d. Vitamin A toxicity

30. Regarding physical activity, adolescents are advised to:
    a. engage in 60 minutes or more of physical activity daily.
    b. spend no more than 3 hours each day watching television.
    c. engage in 30 minutes or more of physical activity daily.
    d. avoid using the computer (other than for homework).

<u>Short Answer Questions</u>

1. Two appropriate primary foods for infants during the first year of life are:

   a.   b.

2. Components of breast milk with immunological benefits include:

   a.   e.

   b.   f.

   c.   g.

   d.

3. Inappropriate formula substitutes for infants include:

   a.   c.

   b.

4. Physical signs of malnutrition in children include:

   a.

   b.

   c.

   d.

   e.

   f.

   g.

   h.

   i.

   j.

5. Signs of food intolerances are:

   a.   f.

   b.   g.

   c.   h.

   d.   i.

   e.

6. Three nutrients that are commonly inadequate in the teenager's diet are:

   a.   c.

   b.

❦ Chapter 16 Answer Key ❧

Summing Up

1. breast milk
2. formula
3. immunological
4. solid
5. same
6. growth
7. retardation
8. subtle
9. behavioral
10. sleep
11. television
12. obesity
13. nutrient-dense
14. activity
15. rapid
16. nutrient
17. calcium

Chapter Study Questions

1. Breast milk is nutritionally tailor-made to meet infant's needs; in fact, for the first 6 months of life, it provides adequate levels of all nutrients except for vitamin D. Breast milk is sterile—meaning it presents no foodborne illness risk—and supplies antibodies and other agents that provide immunological protection, such as oligosaccharides that prevent binding of pathogens; bifidus factors, which promote "friendly" bacterial growth; lactoferrin, which binds iron and makes it unavailable for pathogens; and lactadherin, which inactivates a common virus.

2. To substitute for breast milk occasionally, or to wean to formula during the first year. Formula must meet AAP standards.

3. Physical immaturity; the infant's nutrient needs are met by body stores and formula or breast milk until then. The infant is ready to start eating solid food when he or she is developmentally ready, generally between 4 and 6 months of age. Solids can be begun when the infant's extrusion reflex diminishes, and the ability to swallow nonliquid foods develops. Infants can indicate hunger by leaning towards food with an open mouth, and satiety by turning away or leaning back when food is offered.

4. Cow's milk because it provides insufficient vitamin C and iron and excessive sodium and protein; mixed dinners and heavily sweetened desserts because they are not nutrient dense; sweets of any kind including baby food "desserts" because they convey no nutrients to support growth and may promote obesity; canned vegetables because they contain too much sodium; honey and corn syrup because of the risk of botulism; popcorn, whole grapes, whole beans, hot dog slices, hard candies, and nuts because they can easily choke on these foods.

5. Iron deficiency and possibly vitamin D deficiency. Children should receive 7-10 mg of iron per day. Enough iron-rich foods such as lean meats, fish, poultry, eggs, legumes, and whole or enriched grains to provide this amount should be included in the diet, and milk intake should not be so high as to displace these foods. Vitamin D can be provided by either fortified foods or supplements, in addition to self-synthesis with sun exposure.

6. Nutrient deficiencies manifest in behavioral symptoms. Iron deficiency causes an energy crisis and directly affects moods, attention span, and learning ability. Food additives such as artificial colors and sodium benzoate may exacerbate hyperactivity in children. Television and other "screen time" activities encourage inactivity, and the commercials promote low-nutrient-density foods; excessive television is associated with obesity.

7. A true food allergy is an adverse reaction to foods that involves an immune response (common allergic reactions are skin rash, digestive upset, or respiratory discomfort). Eggs, peanuts, soybeans, and milk are most likely to cause allergy in children; other common causes are tree nuts, wheat, fish, and shellfish. Food allergies can influence a person's nutrition status because excluding allergenic foods (the only treatment) may result in deficiencies of the nutrients those foods normally supply.

8. Obese children are most likely to become obese adults and therefore are at risk for the social, economic and medical ramifications that often accompany obesity. Obese children begin puberty earlier and grow taller than their peers at first, but stop growing at a short height; they display higher levels of total cholesterol, triglycerides, and LDL; they tend to have high blood pressure; they are at risk for diabetes and asthma; they are victims of prejudice. Strategies include modifying dietary and exercise patterns. The initial dietary goal is to reduce the rate of weight gain; that is, to maintain weight while growing in height. Children are encouraged to

eat slowly and select nutrient-dense foods and not be pressured to clean their plates. Daily physical activity should be included. See Table 16-7 (p. 529) for specific recommendations.

9. Parents can allow children to select from healthful choices, to prepare foods, to grow foods in a garden, and to visit food-related places. New foods should be offered one at a time, in small quantities, and at the beginning of the meal, and this should be repeated several times without pressuring the child to accept the food.

10. School lunches can contribute to positive nutrition status if they are nutritious and acceptable. Those that are part of the National School Lunch Program are designed to provide a third of recommended intakes of energy, protein, vitamins A and C, iron, and calcium. The provision of free or low-cost meals may positively impact the nutritional status of children from economically disadvantaged homes.

11. Nutrient needs increase during adolescence because it is a time of growth. Energy needs increase, especially for males, depending on growth rate and activity level. DRI for most vitamins increase, often to adult levels. Iron needs increase to support growth in both genders, to replace menstrual losses in females, and to support lean body mass accretion in males. Calcium requirements peak during this period of bone development. Teenaged girls are more likely to develop iron deficiency because they typically consume fewer iron-rich foods and have lower total energy intakes, resulting in low iron intakes, and because they lose iron during menstruation.

12. Adolescents almost inevitably fall into irregular eating habits. Those who regularly eat meals with their families tend to make more nutrient-dense choices. Adolescents who skip breakfast typically have lower micronutrient intakes and possibly a greater risk of unwanted weight gain. Since snacks provide about a fourth of the average teenager's total daily food energy intake, they can either improve or worsen nutrient intakes depending on whether wholesome (e.g., fresh fruit) or highly processed snack foods are selected. Beverage choices are also important; choosing milk increases calcium intake, whereas soft drinks provide empty and often unneeded kcal.

Key Terms Practice

1. wean
2. lactoferrin
3. adolescence
4. lactadherin
5. colostrum
6. hyperactivity
7. puberty
8. gatekeepers
9. botulism
10. h
11. a
12. g
13. b
14. j
15. f
16. i
17. e
18. d
19. c

Sample Test Questions

1. c (p. 510)
2. b (p. 510)
3. a (pp. 507-508)
4. a (p. 510)
5. e (p. 510)
6. c (p. 513)
7. c (p. 513)
8. b (p. 513)
9. d (p. 517)
10. b (p. 517)
11. a (p. 517)
12. c (p. 519)
13. b (pp. 526-528)
14. a (p. 526)
15. b (p. 524)
16. c (p. 517)
17. a (p. 528)
18. b (p. 537)
19. b (pp. 534-535)
20. d (pp. 527-528)
21. a (p. 531)
22. d (p. 538)
23. c (p. 536)
24. e (pp. 528, 539)
25. a (p. 534)
26. b (pp. 531-532)
27. c (p. 539)
28. c (p. 538)
29. b (p. 522)
30. a (p. 537)

Short Answer Questions

1. breast milk, iron-fortified formula
2. antibodies, oligosaccharides, bifidus factors, lactoferrin, lactadherin, growth factor, enzymes (e.g., lipase)
3. soy beverages, goat's milk, cow's milk
4. See Table 16-6 on p. 522; examples: dull, brittle hair; pale eye membranes; missing and/or discolored teeth, gums bleed easily; flaky facial skin that cracks easily; swollen glands; sore, smooth, purplish tongue; dry, rough skin; spoon-shaped, brittle nails; abnormal heart rate and blood pressure, mental confusion
5. stomachaches, headaches, rapid pulse rate, nausea, wheezing, hives, bronchial irritation, coughs, other related discomforts
6. vitamin D, iron, calcium

⚙ Chapter 17 – Life Cycle Nutrition: ⚙ Adulthood and the Later Years

Chapter Outline

I. Nutrition and Longevity
   A. Observation of Older Adults
      1. Healthy Habits
      2. Physical Activity
   B. Manipulation of Diet
      1. Energy Restriction in Animals
      2. Energy Restriction in Human Beings
II. The Aging Process
   A. Physiological Changes
      1. Body Weight
      2. Body Composition
      3. Immunity and Inflammation
      4. GI Tract
      5. Tooth Loss
      6. Sensory Losses and Other Physical Problems
   B. Other Changes
      1. Psychological Changes
      2. Economic Changes
      3. Social Changes
III. Energy and Nutrient Needs of Older Adults
   A. Water
   B. Energy and Energy Nutrients
      1. Protein
      2. Carbohydrate and Fiber
      3. Fat
   C. Vitamins and Minerals
      1. Vitamin B_{12}
      2. Vitamin D
      3. Folate
      4. Calcium
      5. Iron
      6. Zinc
   D. Nutrient Supplements
IV. Nutrition-Related Concerns of Older Adults

   A. Vision
      1. Cataracts
      2. Macular Degeneration
   B. Arthritis
      1. Osteoarthritis
      2. Rheumatoid Arthritis
      3. Gout
      4. Treatment
   C. The Aging Brain
      1. Nutrient Deficiencies and Brain Function
      2. Alzheimer's Disease
   D. Alcohol
V. Food Choices and Eating Habits of Older Adults
   A. Malnutrition
   B. Food Assistance Programs
   C. Meals for Singles
      1. Foodborne Illness
      2. Spend Wisely
      3. Be Creative
VI. Nutrient-Drug Interactions
   A. The Actions of Drugs
   B. The Interactions between Drugs and Nutrients
      1. Drugs Alter Food Intake
      2. Drugs Alter Nutrient Absorption
      3. Diets Alter Drug Absorption
      4. Drugs Alter Nutrient Metabolism
      5. Diet Alters Drug Metabolism
      6. Drugs Alter Nutrient Excretion
      7. Diets Alter Drug Excretion
      8. Diet-Drug Toxicities
   C. The Inactive Ingredients in Drugs
      1. Sugar, Sorbitol, and Lactose
      2. Sodium

Summing Up

Life expectancy in the United States 1._____ dramatically in the 20th century. Factors that enhance longevity include well-balanced meals, regular 2._____ _____, abstinence from smoking, limited or no 3._____ use, healthy body 4._____, and adequate sleep. Energy restriction in animals seems to 5._____ their lives. Whether such dietary intervention in human beings is beneficial remains 6._____. At the very least, nutrition—especially when combined with regular 7._____ _____—can influence aging and longevity in human beings by supporting good health and preventing 8._____.

Many changes that accompany aging can impair 9._____ status. Among physiological changes, hormone activity alters body 10._____, immune system changes raise the risk of 11._____, atrophic gastritis interferes with digestion and 12._____, and tooth loss limits food choices. Psychological changes such as 13._____, economic changes such as loss of income, and social changes such as 14._____ contribute to poor food intake.

Although some nutrients need special attention in the diet, 15._____ are not routinely recommended. The ever-growing number of older people creates an urgent need to learn more about how their 16._____ requirements differ from those of others and how such knowledge can enhance their 17._____.

Senile dementia and other losses of brain function, including the impaired 18._____ and cognition of alcohol use, afflict millions of older adults, and others face loss of vision due to cataracts or 19._____ _____ or cope with the pain of arthritis. As the number of people older than age 65 continues to grow, the need for 20._____ to these problems becomes urgent. Some problems may be inevitable, but others are preventable and good 21._____ may play a key role.

Older people can benefit from both the nutrients provided and the 22._____ _____ available at congregate meals. Other government programs deliver meals to those who are 23._____- _____. With creativity and careful shopping, those living alone can prepare 24._____, inexpensive meals.

Chapter Study Questions

1. What roles does nutrition play in aging, and what roles can it play in retarding aging?

2. What are some of the physiological changes that occur in the body's systems with aging?

3. Why does the risk of dehydration increase as people age?

4. Why do energy needs usually decline with advancing age?

5. Name some factors that complicate the task of setting nutrient standards for older adults. Which vitamins and minerals need special consideration for the elderly? Explain why.

6. Discuss how nutrition might contribute to or hinder the development of age-related problems associated with vision, the joints, and the brain.

7. What characteristics contribute to malnutrition in older people?

Key Terms Practice

To complete the crossword puzzle, identify the key term that best matches each definition.

Across:
1. Long duration of life.
6. Environmental elements, physical or psychological, that cause stress.
7. Loss of skeletal muscle mass, strength, and quality.
9. Inflammation of a joint, usually accompanied by pain, swelling, and structural changes.
10. Any threat to a person's well-being; a demand placed on the body to adapt.

Down:

2. Nerve cells; the structural and functional units of the nervous system.
3. Clouding of the eye lenses that impairs vision and can lead to blindness.
4. A common form of arthritis characterized by deposits of uric acid crystals in the joints.
5. Difficulty swallowing.
8. Compounds of nitrogen-containing bases such as adenine, guanine, and caffeine.

Match the key terms with their definitions.

11. _____ atrophic gastritis

12. _____ chronological age

13. _____ life expectancy

14. _____ life span

15. _____ macular degeneration

16. _____ physiological age

17. _____ pressure ulcers

18. _____ quality of life

19. _____ stress response

a. the average number of years lived by people in a given society
b. damage to the skin and underlying tissues as a result of compression and poor circulation; commonly seen in people who are bedridden or chair-bound
c. a person's perceived physical and mental well-being
d. a person's age as estimated from her or his body's health and probable life expectancy
e. a person's age in years from his or her date of birth
f. the body's response to stress, mediated by both nerves and hormones
g. the maximum number of years of life attainable by a member of a species
h. a chronic inflammation of the stomach characterized by inadequate hydrochloric acid and intrinsic factor—two key players in vitamin B_{12} absorption
i. deterioration of the macular area of the eye that can lead to loss of central vision and eventual blindness

20. _____ Alzheimer's disease

21. _____ congregate meals

22. _____ Meals on Wheels

23. _____ neurofibrillary tangles

24. _____ osteoarthritis

25. _____ rheumatoid arthritis

26. _____ senile dementia

27. _____ senile plaques

a. a disease of the immune system involving painful inflammation of the joints and related structures
b. a nutrition program that delivers food for the elderly to their homes
c. a degenerative disease of the brain involving memory loss and major structural changes in neuron networks; also known as chronic brain syndrome
d. clumps of the protein fragment beta-amyloid on the nerve cells, commonly found in the brains of people with Alzheimer's dementia
e. snarls of the threadlike strands that extend from the nerve cells, commonly found in the brains of people with Alzheimer's dementia
f. nutrition programs that provide food for the elderly in conveniently located settings such as community centers
g. the loss of brain function beyond the normal loss of physical adeptness and memory that occurs with aging
h. a painful, degenerative disease of the joints that occurs when the cartilage in a joint deteriorates; joint structure is damaged, with loss of function

Sample Test Questions

Select the best answer for each question.

1. The maximum number of years of life attainable by a member of a species is called:
   a. life expectancy.
   b. life span.
   c. longevity.
   d. quality of life.

2. A person's age as estimated from his or her body's health and probable life expectancy is called:
   a. physiological age.
   b. chronological age.
   c. years of healthy life.
   d. longevity.

3. What is the life expectancy for black males and females in the U.S.?
   a. 71 years for males, 77 years for females
   b. 76 years for males, 81 years for females
   c. 79 years for males, 84 years for females
   d. 85 years for males, 89 years for females

4. What is the life expectancy for white males and females in the U.S.?
   a. 71 years for males, 77 years for females
   b. 76 years for males, 81 years for females
   c. 79 years for males, 84 years for females
   d. 85 years for males, 89 years for females

5. Studies of adults show that longevity is enhanced, in part, by all of the following **except**:
   a. weight control.
   b. not smoking.
   c. short periods of sleep.
   d. no or moderate alcohol intake.

6. What would be the physiological age of a 75-year-old woman whose physical health is equivalent to that of her 50-year-old daughter?
   a. 25 years
   b. 50 years
   c. 75 years
   d. 125 years

7. A person's perceived physical and mental well-being is called:
   a. longevity.
   b. life expectancy.
   c. life span.
   d. quality of life.

8. Environmental elements that cause the body to adapt are:
   a. stress responses.
   b. fight-or-flight hormones.
   c. stressors.
   d. eustress.

9. Which of the following has been associated with regular physical activity in older adults?
   a. Retention of sodium
   b. Increase in blood LDL
   c. Increased death rates
   d. Improved quality of life

10. Which of the following tends to decline with aging?
    a. Body fat
    b. Muscle mass
    c. Blood lipids
    d. Blood pressure

11. Which of the following statements is true regarding exercise and older people?
    a. Regular physical activity provides a minimal benefit to older people.
    b. Older people should not engage in strength training.
    c. Physical activity may help older people maintain their independence.
    d. Loss of muscle mass is an inevitable part of aging.

12. Which of the following statements is true regarding energy restriction and aging?
    a. Energy restriction of 30% extends human life and should be encouraged.
    b. There is no evidence that energy restriction is beneficial for older people.
    c. An energy restriction of 10-20% lowers body fat and blood pressure.
    d. Fasting for several days consecutively appears to be beneficial.

13. As people age, they often experience:
    a. declining immune system function.
    b. loss of elasticity of intestinal walls.
    c. tooth loss.
    d. All of the above
    e. a and b

14. Loss of skeletal muscle mass, strength, and quality that often occurs with aging is called:
    a. dysphagia.
    b. hypertrophy.
    c. sarcopenia.
    d. sarcoma.

15. Dysphagia, which occurs most often among the elderly, is described as:
    a. difficulty chewing.
    b. difficulty swallowing.
    c. difficulty digesting.
    d. difficulty eliminating.

16. Atrophic gastritis is a condition that can especially impair the absorption of:
    a. vitamin B$_{12}$ and biotin.
    b. calcium and iron.
    c. glucose and amino acids.
    d. All of the above
    e. a and b

17. Studies of the eating habits of older adults demonstrate all of the following **except**:
    a. those who live alone in federally funded housing have higher-quality diets.
    b. adults living alone often consume insufficient amounts of food.
    c. malnutrition is associated with a lower level of education.
    d. only about one in three who are SNAP eligible participate.

18. Nutrient needs of older people:
    a. vary from individual to individual and show pronounced differences.
    b. increase; therefore, supplementation is required.
    c. remain the same as in young adult life.
    d. decrease.

19. Which of the following is a feature of elderly people and water balance?
    a. They do not seem to feel thirsty or recognize dryness of the mouth.
    b. They have a higher total body water content compared with younger adults.
    c. They show increased frequency of urination, which results in higher requirements.
    d. They frequently show symptoms of overhydration such as mental lapses and disorientation.

20. Because energy needs decrease with age, healthy elderly people should obtain protein from:
    a. liquid nutritional formulas.
    b. only vegan diets.
    c. fried chicken with gravy.
    d. low-kcalorie sources of high-quality protein.

21. To avoid constipation, older adults should:
    a. eat high-fiber foods and drink plenty of water.
    b. consume refined carbohydrate-containing foods.
    c. stop taking prescribed medications.
    d. eat only raw foods.

22. Which of the following statements describes one aspect of mineral nutrition of older adults?
    a. Zinc intake is adequate for about 95% of this group.
    b. Calcium intakes of females are near the RDA for this group.
    c. Iron-deficiency anemia in this population group is less common than in younger adults.
    d. Calcium allowances for this group have recently been decreased by the DRI Committee.

23. What condition is characterized by clouding of the lenses of the eye that impairs vision, especially in the elderly?
    a. Macular degeneration
    b. Cataracts
    c. Retinitis
    d. Carotenoids

24. What nutrients may be protective against cataract formation?
    a. Iron and calcium
    b. Chromium and zinc
    c. Vitamin B$_{12}$ and folate
    d. Vitamin C and vitamin E

25. What dietary components may be protective against macular degeneration?
    a. Calcium
    b. DHA
    c. Lutein
    d. a and b
    e. b and c

26. There is an established connection between osteoarthritis and:
    a. calcium.
    b. vitamin D.
    c. omega-3 fatty acids.
    d. overweight.

208

27. How is nutrition linked to rheumatoid arthritis?
    a. The immune system relies on adequate nutrition.
    b. Omega-3 fatty acids may reduce joint tenderness.
    c. Rheumatoid arthritis is promoted by obesity.
    d. None of the above

28. Clumps of beta-amyloid on the nerve cells are called:
    a. gout.
    b. senile plaques.
    c. neurofibrillary tangles.
    d. neurons.

29. Goals of the federal OAA Nutrition Program include the provision of all of the following **except**:
    a. transportation services.
    b. high-cost nutritious meals.
    c. opportunities for social interaction.
    d. counseling and referral to other social services.

30. To avoid foodborne illness, older people should:
    a. only eat raw foods.
    b. not eat or drink unpasteurized milk or milk products.
    c. not eat undercooked eggs, meat, poultry or fish.
    d. a and b
    e. b and c

Short Answer Questions

1. Three commonly used age groups for older people are:
    a.
    c.
    b.

2. Six lifestyle behaviors that seem to have the greatest influence on people's health and therefore on their physiological age are:
    a.
    b.
    c.
    d.
    e.
    f.

3. Five potential positive outcomes of reducing energy intake by 10 to 20% are:
    a.
    d.
    b.
    e.
    c.

4. Two changes in the immune system associated with aging and responsible for chronic inflammation are:
    a.
    b.

5. Five consequences of atrophic gastritis are:
    a.
    d.
    b.
    e.
    c.

6. Six conditions requiring dental care:

a.   d.

b.   e.

c.   f.

7. Three non-physiological factors that play major roles in a person's ability and willingness to eat are:

a.   c.

b.

8. Six micronutrients of particular concern to the elderly are:

a.   d.

b.   e.

c.   f.

9. Four risk factors for osteoarthritis are:

a.   c.

b.   d.

10. Four factors that protect brain function are:

a.   c.

b.   d.

11. Seven ways that malnutrition limits a person's ability to function and diminishes quality of life are:

a.   e.

b.   f.

c.   g.

d.

❧ Chapter 17 Answer Key ❧

Summing Up

1. increased
2. physical activity
3. alcohol
4. weight
5. lengthen
6. unknown
7. physical activity
8. disease
9. nutrition
10. composition
11. infections
12. absorption
13. depression
14. loneliness
15. supplements
16. nutrient
17. health
18. memory
19. macular degeneration
20. solutions
21. nutrition
22. social interaction
23. home-bound
24. nutritious

Chapter Study Questions

1. Nutrition can slow some aspects of the aging process within the natural limits set by heredity. Eating well-balanced meals on a regular basis and limiting or avoiding alcohol consumption are 2 of the 6 lifestyle behaviors that seem to have the greatest influence on physiological age (age as estimated based on health and probable life expectancy). Extreme energy restriction in humans is problematic, but moderate restrictions in energy intake (10-20%) often result in favorable metabolic changes that can reduce chronic disease risk. Oxidative damage (which is thought to contribute to aging) can be reduced by a diet abundant in fruits, vegetables, olive oil, and moderate amounts of red wine, which supply antioxidant phytochemicals.

2. Energy needs decrease; and older people tend to gain body fat and lose muscle mass. Hormone activity alters body composition, immune system changes raise the risk of infections, atrophic gastritis interferes with digestion and absorption, and tooth loss limits food choices. Sensory losses can interfere with the selection, acquisition, preparation, and enjoyment of foods. Depression, economics, and social changes resulting in loneliness contribute to poor food intake.

3. Risk of dehydration increases as people age because total body water volume declines (smaller losses are required to result in dehydration), and many older people do not feel thirsty or notice mouth dryness. Poor mobility may limit access to fluids or result in a reluctance to drink much because of the diuretic effect.

4. Energy needs usually decline with advancing age because lean body mass diminishes, reducing basal metabolic rate. As people age they may reduce their physical activity, promoting loss of lean mass and further lowering energy needs.

5. Some vitamin and mineral needs remain constant from early adulthood to later years; however, the nutrition needs of people 51 to 70 differ from those of adults over 70. Individual differences become more pronounced as people grow older. The effects of chronic diseases and various medications influence nutrient needs. Older adults must pay special attention to vitamin B_{12}, vitamin D, folate, calcium, iron, and zinc. Atrophic gastritis (in ~10-30% of adults >50) reduces hydrochloric acid and intrinsic factor secretion, inhibiting vitamin B_{12} digestion and absorption. Vitamin D deficiency is possible because many adults drink little or no milk, and skin synthesis and kidney activation of the vitamin decline with age. The elderly often have conditions or take medications that compromise folate status. Iron-deficiency anemia is less common in older adults, but may develop in those with low intakes, diseases or medical treatments causing blood loss, or poor absorption due to atrophic gastritis or antacid use. Zinc intake is commonly low in this population, and some medications impair its absorption or increase its excretion.

6. Oxidative stress plays a role in cataract development and macular degeneration. Antioxidant nutrients may help minimize the damage; consuming adequate intakes of vitamins C and E and carotenoids may help cataracts reduce risk or slow progression. Supplements of DHA, some B vitamins, and carotenoids may help prevent macular degeneration. Being overweight aggravates osteoarthritis partly because weight-bearing joints have to carry excess poundage. Weight loss may relieve some of this pain. Some individuals with rheumatoid arthritis may experience some relief when they consume a diet of fatty fish, vegetables, and olive oil, which may moderate the inflammatory response. Since rheumatoid arthritis involves oxidative damage to joints, antioxidants (vitamins C and E, carotenoids) may also prevent or relieve pain. Gout may be prevented by lowering uric acid levels by limiting intakes of alcohol, meat, seafood, and sugar-sweetened beverages. Nutrient

deficiencies may contribute to age-related loss of memory and cognition; thus, diet and exercise may prevent, slow, or reduce these losses. Middle-age overweight/obesity is associated with development of dementia, particularly Alzheimer's, as is oxidative stress. Heart-healthy diets including DHA may promote brain health. Chronic alcohol use contributes to memory and cognition impairments.

7. Physically, older people may not be mobile and thus may be unable to purchase and prepare nutritious meals. Psychologically, many older people live alone and may not prepare food for one; financially, many live on social security and have a limited income. Additional risk factors for malnutrition include disease, poor eating habits, tooth loss or mouth pain, reduced social contact, multiple medication use, involuntary weight changes, and advanced age (>80).

Key Terms Practice

1. longevity
2. neurons
3. cataracts
4. gout
5. dysphagia
6. stressors
7. sarcopenia
8. purines
9. arthritis
10. stress
11. h
12. e
13. a
14. g
15. i
16. d
17. b
18. c
19. f
20. c
21. f
22. b
23. e
24. h
25. a
26. g
27. d

Sample Test Questions

1. b (p. 552)
2. a (p. 553)
3. a (p. 552)
4. b (p. 552)
5. c (p. 553)
6. b (p. 553)
7. d (p. 553)
8. c (p. 556)
9. d (p. 553)
10. b (p. 557)
11. c (p. 554)
12. c (p. 556)
13. d (pp. 557-558)
14. c (p. 557)
15. b (p. 558)
16. e (p. 558)
17. a (pp. 559-560)
18. a (p. 560)
19. a (p. 560)
20. d (p. 561)
21. a (p. 561)
22. c (p. 562)
23. b (p. 564)
24. d (p. 564)
25. e (p. 564)
26. d (p. 564)
27. b (p. 565)
28. b (p. 566)
29. b (p. 569-570)
30. e (p. 570)

Short Answer Questions

1. young old (65–74 years), old old (75–84 years), oldest old (≥85 years).
2. eating well-balanced meals (rich in fruits, vegetables, whole grains, poultry, fish, and low fat milk products); engaging in physical activity regularly; not smoking; not using alcohol, or using it in moderation; maintaining a healthy body weight; sleeping regularly and adequately
3. lower body weight, reduced body fat, lower blood pressure, improved blood lipids, enhanced insulin response
4. loss of function, overstimulation in response to illness
5. inflamed stomach, increased bacterial growth, reduced hydrochloric acid, reduced intrinsic factor, increased risk of nutrient deficiencies (notably of vitamin B_{12})
6. dry mouth; eating difficulty; lack of dental care within past 2 years; tooth or mouth pain; altered food selections; lesions, sores, or lumps in mouth
7. psychological changes (such as depression), economic changes (such as loss of income), social changes (such as loneliness)
8. vitamin B_{12}, vitamin D, folate, calcium, iron, zinc
9. age, smoking, high BMI at age 40, lack of hormone therapy (in women)
10. physical activities, intellectual challenges, social interactions, a balanced diet rich in antioxidants
11. impairing muscle function, decreasing bone mass, limiting immune defenses, reducing cognitive abilities, delaying wound healing, slowing recovery from surgery, increasing hospitalizations

❧ Chapter 18 – Diet and Health ❧

Chapter Outline

I.   Nutrition and Infectious Diseases
   A.   The Immune System
      1.   Phagocytes: Neutrophils and Macrophages
      2.   Lymphocytes: B-cells
      3.   Lymphocytes: T-cells
   B.   Nutrition and Immunity
   C.   HIV and AIDS
   D.   Inflammation and Chronic Diseases
II. Nutrition and Chronic Diseases
III. Cardiovascular Disease
   A.   How Atherosclerosis Develops
      1.   Inflammation
      2.   Plaques
      3.   Blood Clots
      4.   Blood Pressure
      5.   The Result: Heart Attacks and Strokes
   B.   Risk Factors for Coronary Heart Disease
      1.   Age, Gender, and Family History
      2.   High LDL and Low HDL Cholesterol
      3.   High Blood Pressure (Hypertension)
      4.   Diabetes
      5.   Obesity and Physical Inactivity
      6.   Cigarette Smoking
      7.   Atherogenic Diet
      8.   Other Risk Factors
      9.   Metabolic Syndrome
   C.   Recommendations for Reducing Coronary Heart Disease Risk
      1.   Cholesterol Screening
      2.   Lifestyle Changes
IV. Hypertension
   A.   How Hypertension Develops
   B.   Risk Factors for Hypertension
   C.   Treatment of Hypertension
      1.   Weight Control
      2.   Physical Activity
      3.   The DASH Diet
      4.   Salt/Sodium Intake
      5.   Medications
V.   Diabetes Mellitus

   A.   How Diabetes Develops
      1.   Type 1 Diabetes
      2.   Type 2 Diabetes
   B.   Complications of Diabetes
      1.   Diseases of the Large Blood Vessels
      2.   Diseases of the Small Blood Vessels
      3.   Diseases of the Nerves
   C.   Recommendations for Diabetes
      1.   Total Carbohydrate Intake
      2.   Carbohydrate Sources
      3.   Dietary Fat
      4.   Protein
      5.   Alcohol
      6.   Recommendations for Type 1 Diabetes
      7.   Recommendations for Type 2 Diabetes
VI. Cancer
   A.   How Cancer Develops
      1.   Environmental Factors
      2.   Dietary Factors—Cancer Initiators
      3.   Dietary Factors—Cancer Promoters
      4.   Dietary Factors—Antipromoters
   B.   Recommendations for Reducing Cancer Risks
VII. Recommendations for Chronic Diseases
   A.   Recommendations for the Population
   B.   Recommendations for Individuals
   C.   Recommendations for Each Individual
VIII. Complementary and Alternative Medicine
   A.   Defining Complementary and Alternative Medicine
   B.   Sound Research, Loud Controversy
      1.   Placebo Effect
      2.   Risks versus Benefits
   C.   Nutrition-Related Alternative Therapies
      1.   Foods
      2.   Vitamin and Mineral Supplements
      3.   Herbal Remedies
      4.   Herbal Precautions
   D.   Internet Precautions
   E.   The Consumer's Perspective

Summing Up

Public health measures such as purification of 1._____ and safe handling of food help prevent the spread of 2._____ in developed nations, and immunizations and antibiotics protect individuals. Nevertheless, some infectious diseases still endanger people today. Nutrition cannot prevent or cure infectious diseases, but adequate intakes of all the nutrients can help support the 3._____ system as the body defends against disease-causing agents. If the immune system is impaired because of 4._____ or diseases such as AIDS, a person becomes 5._____ to infectious disease.

6._____ underlies many chronic diseases.

7._____ _____ and cancers are the two leading causes of death in the United States, and strokes and 8._____ also rank among the top 10. All four of these chronic diseases have significant links with 9._____. Other lifestyle risk factors and genetics are also important.

Atherosclerosis is characterized by plaque build-up in 10._____ walls. Plaques rupturing or blood clotting can cause heart attacks and 11._____. Quitting 12._____ and engaging in regular 13._____ _____ improve heart health.

The most effective dietary strategy for preventing hypertension is 14._____ control. Also beneficial are diets rich in fruits, vegetables, nuts, and low-fat milk products and low in fat, saturated fat, and 15._____.

Diabetes is characterized by high blood 16._____ and either insufficient 17._____, ineffective insulin, or a combination of the two. People with type 1 diabetes coordinate diet, 18._____, and physical activity to help control their blood glucose. Those with type 2 diabetes benefit most from a diet and physical activity program that controls glucose fluctuations and promotes 19._____ loss.

Some dietary factors, such as 20._____ and heavily smoked foods, may initiate cancer development; others, such as animal fats, may 21._____ cancer once it has gotten started; and still others, such as fiber, antioxidant nutrients, and phytochemicals, may act as 22._____ that protect against the development of cancer. By eating many fruits, 23._____, legumes, and whole grains and reducing 24._____ _____ intake, people obtain the best possible nutrition at the lowest possible risk. Minimizing 25._____ _____ through regular physical activity and a healthy diet is also beneficial.

Clearly, optimal nutrition plays a key role in keeping people healthy and reducing the risk of 26._____ diseases. To have the greatest impact possible, dietary recommendations are aimed at the entire 27._____, not just at the individuals who might benefit most. Recommendations focus on 28._____ control and urge people to limit saturated and 29._____ fat; increase fiber-rich fruits, vegetables, and 30._____ _____; and balance 31._____ intake with physical activity. A person can do no better than to incorporate those suggestions into his or her daily life.

Chapter Study Questions

1. List the major types of blood cells involved in the immune response, and briefly describe their roles.

2. What is HIV infection? What are the consequences of HIV infection? Is this disease related to nutrition?

214

3. Discuss the relationship between nutrition and chronic diseases.

4. Identify the major diet-related risk factors for atherosclerosis, hypertension, cancer, and type 2 diabetes.

5. Describe some ways in which people can alter their lifestyles to lower their risk of CHD.

6. Describe some steps that people with hypertension can take to lower their blood pressure.

7. Name the two major types of diabetes and describe some differences between them. How do dietary recommendations for each type of diabetes compare with the recommendations for healthy people?

8. Differentiate among cancer initiators, promoters, and antipromoters. Which nutrients or foods fit into each of these categories?

9. Describe the characteristics of a diet that might offer the best protection against the onset of cancer.

10. Summarize dietary recommendations to prevent chronic diseases.

Key Terms Practice

To complete the crossword puzzle, identify the key term that best matches each definition.

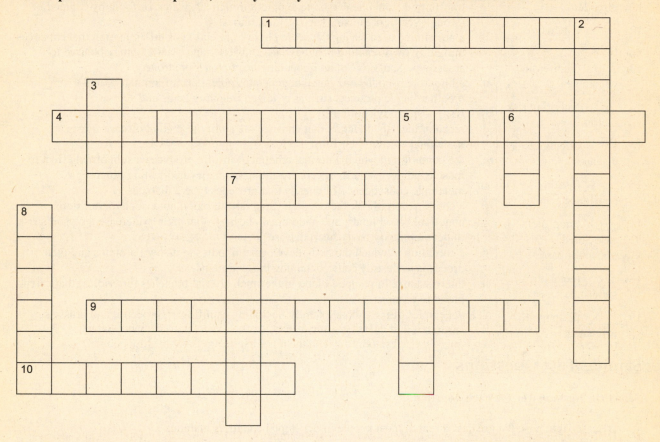

Across:
1. The formation of a blood clot that may obstruct a blood vessel, causing gradual tissue death.
4. Disorders of the small blood vessels.
7. A painful feeling of tightness or pressure in and around the heart, often radiating to the back, neck, and arms; caused by a lack of oxygen to an area of heart muscle.
9. Elevated blood glucose concentrations.
10. The obstruction of a blood vessel by a traveling clot, causing sudden tissue death.

Down:
2. Multiple factors operating together in such a way that their combined effects are greater than the sum of their individual effects.
3. The late stage of HIV infection, in which severe complications develop.
5. Tiny, disc-shaped bodies in the blood, important in blood clot formation.
6. The virus that causes an infection that progresses to become an immune system disorder that leaves its victims defenseless against numerous infections.
7. An abnormal enlargement or bulging of a blood vessel (usually an artery) caused by damage to or weakness in the blood vessel wall.
8. An event in which the blood flow to a part of the brain is cut off; also called cerebrovascular accident (CVA).

Match the key terms with their definitions.

11. _____ autoimmune disorder

12. _____ C-reactive protein

13. _____ cruciferous vegetables

14. _____ emerging risk factors

15. _____ infectious diseases

16. _____ insulin resistance

17. _____ lipoprotein-associated phospholipase

18. _____ metabolic syndrome

19. _____ peripheral resistance

a. diseases caused by bacteria, viruses, parasites, or other microorganisms that can be transmitted from one person to another through air, water, or food; by contact; or through vector organisms such as mosquitoes

b. a protein released during the acute phase of infection or inflammation that enhances immunity by promoting phagocytosis and activating platelets; may be used to assess a person's risk of an impending heart attack or stroke

c. a lipoprotein-bound enzyme that generates potent proinflammatory and proatherogenic products such as oxidized free fatty acids and lysophosphatidylcholine

d. recently identified factors that enhance the ability to predict disease risk in an individual

e. the condition in which a normal amount of insulin produces a subnormal effect in muscle, adipose, and liver cells, resulting in an elevated fasting glucose; a metabolic consequence of obesity that precedes type 2 diabetes

f. a combination of risk factors—elevated fasting blood glucose, hypertension, abnormal blood lipids, and abdominal obesity—that greatly increase a person's risk of developing coronary heart disease

g. a condition in which the body develops antibodies to its own proteins and then proceeds to destroy cells containing these proteins

h. the resistance to pumped blood in the small arterial branches (arterioles) that carry blood to tissues

i. vegetables of the cabbage family, including cauliflower, broccoli, and brussels sprouts

Sample Test Questions

Select the best answer for each question.

1. Diseases that pose the greatest threat to most people in developed countries include:
   1. tuberculosis.
   2. smallpox.
   3. diseases of the heart and blood vessels.
   4. cancer.
   5. diabetes.

   a. 1, 2, 3
   b. 2, 3, 4
   c. 3, 4, 5
   d. 1, 3, 5

2. Which disease has some relationship with nutrition?
   a. Cancer
   b. Diabetes
   c. Heart disease
   d. a and b
   e. a, b, and c

3. What body system usually defends the body against infectious diseases?
   a. Central nervous system
   b. Inflammation
   c. Immune system
   d. Autoimmune system

4. What is the body's first line of defense against infection?
   a. Skin and mucous membranes
   b. T-cells
   c. B-cells
   d. All of the above

5. Organs of the immune system include the:
   a. heart.
   b. spleen.
   c. thymus.
   d. a and b
   e. b and c

6. Cells of the immune system include:
   a. phagocytes.
   b. lymphocytes.
   c. B-cells.
   d. a and c
   e. a, b, and c

7. What proteins are secreted by phagocytes to activate the immune response?
   a. Neutrophils
   b. Cytokines
   c. Macrophages
   d. T-cells

8. What type of cells produce antibodies in response to infection?
   a. B-cells
   b. T-cells
   c. Platelets
   d. Immunoglobulins

9. Inflammation:
   a. is beneficial when acute.
   b. is beneficial when chronic.
   c. causes the symptoms of AIDS.
   d. is preventable through good nutrition.

10. _____ and _____ create a synergistic downward spiral.
    a. Disease, wellness
    b. Disease, malnutrition
    c. HIV, obesity
    d. HIV, AIDS

11. Which of the following statements is true regarding HIV/AIDS?
    a. AIDS prevention depends on good nutrition.
    b. A cure has been developed for HIV/AIDS.
    c. HIV is transmitted by direct contact with contaminated body fluids.
    d. In the U.S., the death rate from AIDS has increased since the 1990s.

12. Being obese increases the probability of developing which of the following?
    a. Cancer
    b. Hypertension
    c. Diabetes
    d. Atherosclerosis
    e. All of the above

13. Mounds of lipid material mixed up with smooth muscle cells and connective tissue that develop in the artery walls are called:
    a. osteoporosis.
    b. atherosclerosis.
    c. CVD.
    d. plaques.

14. The immunological response to tissue damage involved with atherosclerosis is called:
    a. hyperglycemia.
    b. hypoglycemia.
    c. inflammation.
    d. irritation.

15. Which of the following is released during the acute phase of inflammation and activates platelets?
    a. C-reactive protein
    b. Plaques
    c. Cholesterol
    d. Macrophages

16. The event in which an embolus lodges in vessels that feed the heart muscle, causing sudden tissue death, is called a:
    a. thrombus.
    b. heart attack.
    c. stroke.
    d. transient ischemic attack.

17. Damage that occurs when the blood vessels carrying blood to the heart become narrow and occluded is called:
    a. an aneurysm.
    b. a plaque.
    c. an aorta.
    d. coronary heart disease.

18. Which two conditions worsen each other?
    a. Cancer, diverticulosis
    b. Cancer, diabetes
    c. Hypertension, atherosclerosis
    d. Hypoglycemia, hypertension

19. Risk factors for atherosclerosis that can be minimized by behavior change include:
    1. smoking.
    2. hypertension.
    3. gender.
    4. lack of exercise.
    5. obesity.
    6. heredity.
    7. high LDL.

    a. 1, 2, 3, 4, 5
    b. 1, 2, 4, 5, 6
    c. 2, 3, 4, 5, 7
    d. 1, 2, 4, 5, 7

20. A condition in which the body develops antibodies to its own proteins and then destroys cells containing these proteins is called:
    a. an inflammation disorder.
    b. AIDS.
    c. hyperglycemia.
    d. an autoimmune disorder.

21. A cluster of risk factors including low HDL, high blood pressure, insulin resistance, and abdominal obesity is known as:
    a. emerging risk factors.
    b. metabolic syndrome.
    c. peripheral resistance.
    d. an autoimmune disorder.

22. When the pancreas loses its ability to synthesize insulin and then hyperglycemia develops, this is called:
    a. type 1 diabetes.
    b. type 2 diabetes.
    c. prediabetes.
    d. hyperlipidemia.

23. Diseases that result from the unchecked growth of malignant tumors are:
    a. AIDS.
    b. cancers.
    c. hypertension.
    d. autoimmune disorders.

24. A _____ diet is linked to colon cancer development.
    a. high-red meat
    b. low-fat
    c. high-fiber
    d. high-food additive

25. What term indicates that cancer has spread to other parts of the body?
    a. Malignant
    b. Benign
    c. Promoter
    d. Metastasize

26. What term refers to dietary factors that start cancer development?
    a. Promoters
    b. Initiators
    c. Antipromoters
    d. Cruciferous

27. To inhibit cancer promotion,
    a. consume high-protein and high-fat diets.
    b. reduce saturated and *trans* fat intakes.
    c. increase omega-3 fatty acid intake.
    d. a and b
    e. b and c

28. Dietary antipromoters include:
    a. fruits and vegetables.
    b. grilled meats.
    c. refined breads.
    d. B vitamins.

29. Recommendations for reducing chronic disease risk include:
    a. take multivitamin/mineral supplements daily.
    b. increase fat intake.
    c. severely restrict kcalories.
    d. achieve and maintain a healthy body weight.

30. Health recommendations that urge dietary changes only for people who are known to need them are taking a:
    a. preventive approach.   c. secondary approach.
    b. population approach.   d. medical approach.

Short Answer Questions

1. Four public health measures that protect people from infection are:
   a.   c.
   b.   d.

2. Eleven nutrients known to affect immunity are:
   a.   g.
   b.   h.
   c.   i.
   d.   j.
   e.   k.
   f.

3. Four of the 10 leading causes of death in the U.S. that have significant links with nutrition are:
   a.   c.
   b.   d.

4. Four major sources of omega-3 fatty acids include:
   a.   c.
   b.   d.

5. Eleven strategies to reduce risk of CHD are:
   a.
   b.
   c.
   d.
   e.
   f.
   g.
   h.
   i.
   j.
   k.

6. The five possible criteria for metabolic syndrome are:

   a.

   b.

   c.

   d.

   e.

7. Five risk factors for hypertension are:

   a.   d.

   b.   e.

   c.

8. Three things that must be coordinated in order to manage type 1 diabetes are:

   a.   c.

   b.

9. The 3 steps in cancer development are:

   a.

   b.

   c.

⑥ Chapter 18 Answer Key ⑥

Summing Up

1. water	9. nutrition	16. insulin	25. weight gain
2. infection	10. artery	18. insulin	26. chronic
3. immune	11. strokes	19. weight	27. population
4. malnutrition	12. smoking	20. alcohol	28. weight
5. vulnerable	13. physical activity	21. promote	29. *trans*
6. Inflammation	14. weight	22. antipromoters	30. whole grains
7. Heart disease	15. sodium	23. vegetables	31. food
8. diabetes	15. glucose	24. saturated fat	

Chapter Study Questions

1. Two types of white blood cells that participate in immunity are phagocytes and lymphocytes. Phagocytes (neutrophils and macrophages) engulf and digest pathogens and secrete cytokines to activate metabolic and immune responses to infection. There are two types of lymphocytes: B-cells, which produce antibodies, and T-cells, which directly attack invaders that display specific antigens on their surfaces by releasing chemicals.

2. HIV infection is infection with the human immunodeficiency virus; it attacks the immune system and causes those who are infected to be vulnerable to opportunistic infections. Development of this incurable disease is completely unrelated to nutrition. Rather, it is caused by exposure to infected body fluids such as blood, semen, or vaginal secretions, and is not preventable or treatable with diet. An adequate diet may improve responses to drug treatment, shorten hospital stays, and increase independence and quality of life; careful attention to food safety can minimize exposure to foodborne opportunistic infections.

3. Four of the ten leading causes of death in the U. S. have some relationship with diet. Single nutrients can affect single diseases (e.g., calcium and osteoporosis, saturated fat and heart disease). Also, each nutrient may have connections with several diseases because its role in the body is not specific to a disease, but to a body function. Obesity, which results from overnutrition, promotes several leading chronic diseases. Attention to nutrition may prevent some chronic diseases, or may improve the quality of life and slow disease progression.

4. Specific diet-related risk factors are: diets high in salty or pickled foods (hypertension and cancer), high-saturated/*trans* fat diets (all four), low intake of high-fiber and -phytochemical foods like fruits/vegetables (atherosclerosis, cancer, and diabetes), low vitamin and/or mineral intakes (atherosclerosis, hypertension, and cancer), and excessive alcohol consumption (atherosclerosis, hypertension, and cancer). A high added sugar intake from sweetened beverages may promote obesity, which is associated with all four.

5. Maintain appropriate body weight, exercise regularly, and do not smoke. To control blood cholesterol, consume a diet high in fiber- and potassium-rich vegetables and fruits with less than 7% of total kcal from saturated fat, less than 1% of total kcal from *trans* fat, and less than 300 mg/day of cholesterol. Consume fatty fish rich in omega-3 fatty acids and soy foods in place of high-fat animal foods. Dietary soluble fiber and plant sterols/stanols can improve blood lipids. Minimize added sugar intake, limit sodium to 1500/day or less, and consume alcohol in moderation (if at all).

6. Balance energy intake and output to maintain appropriate body weight (or lose weight if overweight), lower salt intake, exercise regularly, eat adequate amounts of calcium and potassium, lower saturated/*trans* fat intake, and, if you drink alcohol, do so in moderation. Follow the DASH (Dietary Approaches to Stop Hypertension) diet, which is rich in fruits, vegetables, nuts, and low-fat milk products and is low in fat and saturated fat.

7. Two types of diabetes are type 1 and type 2. In type 1 (an autoimmune disorder) the person produces no insulin; type 2 is more common and is associated with obesity and insulin resistance. Nutrition therapy focuses on maintaining optimal nutrition status, controlling blood glucose, achieving a desirable lipid profile, controlling blood pressure, and preventing and treating the complications of diabetes. Distributing carbohydrate intake so it is consistent throughout the day is a key strategy. General dietary guidelines for good health are similar to meal planning for diabetes; the major difference is that the amount and timing of carbohydrate intake must be controlled in diabetes to maintain normal blood glucose levels, especially in those who take insulin.

8. Initiators are factors such as carcinogens that alter the genetic material responsible for controlling cell division. Promoters enhance cancer development once it has begun; antipromoters oppose cancer development. Initiators: alcohol, fried/broiled meat, grilled foods, red and processed meats, and fried potatoes. Promoters: possibly high-fat foods, especially animal fats. Antipromoters: high-fiber foods, garlic, milk, calcium, nonstarchy and allum vegetables, fruits, beta-carotene/lycopene and other carotenoids (from foods), vitamin C (from foods), folate (from foods), and selenium.

9. A diet for cancer prevention provides sufficient energy to maintain as lean a body composition as possible within the normal BMI range; this can be accomplished in part by limiting intake of energy-dense foods and sweetened beverages. It consists primarily of plant foods such as varied nonstarchy vegetables, fruits, unprocessed grains, and legumes. It includes <18 oz./week of red meat, no processed meats, little or no alcohol, and few salted foods (<6 g salt/day). Moldy grains or legumes are omitted.

10. Recommendations focus on weight control and urge people to maintain a healthy weight; increase physical activity; moderate total fat limit saturated and *trans* fat; increase fiber-rich fruits, vegetables, and whole grains; reduce added sugars and sodium; and consume alcohol in moderation (if at all).

Key Terms Practice

1. thrombosis
2. synergistic
3. AIDS
4. microangiopathies
5. platelets
6. HIV
7. A: angina, D: aneurysm
8. stroke
9. hyperglycemia
10. embolism
11. g
12. b
13. i
14. d
15. a
16. e
17. c
18. f
19. h

Sample Test Questions

1. c (p. 581)
2. e (p. 585)
3. c (p. 582)
4. a (p. 582)
5. e (p. 582)
6. e (p. 583)
7. b (p. 583)
8. a (p. 583)
9. a (p. 584)
10. b (p. 584)
11. c (p. 584)
12. e (p. 586)
13. d (p. 587)
14. c (p. 587)
15. a (p. 587)
16. b (p. 587)
17. d (p. 587)
18. c (p. 590)
19. d (pp. 589-590)
20. d (p. 598)
21. b (p. 591)
22. a (p. 598)
23. b (p. 602)
24. a (p. 605)
25. d (pp. 602-603)
26. b (p. 603)
27. e (p. 605-606)
28. a (pp. 604, 605)
29. d (p. 607)
30. d (p. 608)

Short Answer Questions

1. purification of water, safe handling of food, immunizations, antibiotics
2. fatty acids, folate, iron, protein, selenium, vitamin A, vitamin B$_6$, vitamin C, vitamin D, vitamin E, zinc
3. heart disease, cancers, strokes, diabetes mellitus
4. vegetable oils (canola, soybean, flaxseed), walnuts, flaxseeds, fatty fish (mackerel, salmon, sardines)
5. achieve and maintain a healthy body weight; limit saturated fat, *trans* fat, and cholesterol; choose a diet rich in foods high in soluble fibers; choose a diet high in potassium-rich foods and low in sodium; minimize intake of beverages and foods with added sugars; consume fatty fish rich in omega-3 fatty acids (salmon, tuna, sardines) at least twice a week; consume food products that contain added plant sterols or stanols; consume soy foods to replace animal and dairy products that contain saturated fat and cholesterol; if alcohol is consumed, limit it to one drink daily for women and two drinks daily for men; participate in at least 30 minutes of moderate-intensity endurance activity on most days of the week; minimize exposure to any form of tobacco or tobacco smoke
6. abdominal obesity; triglycerides ≥150 mg/dL; HDL <40 mg/dL in men or <50 mg/dL in women; blood pressure ≥130/85 mm Hg; fasting blood glucose ≥100 mg/dL
7. aging, genetics, obesity, salt sensitivity, alcohol
8. diet, physical activity, insulin
9. a. Initiation – genetic (DNA) mutation in a cell induces abnormal cell division
   b. Promotion – promoters enhance the development of abnormal cells, resulting in tumor formation
   c. Metastasis – release of abnormal cells by the tumor into the circulatory system

❧ Chapter 19 – Consumer Concerns ❧
about Foods and Water

Chapter Outline

I. Foodborne Illnesses
   A. Foodborne Infections and Food Intoxications
     1. Foodborne Infections
     2. Food Intoxications
   B. Food Safety in the Marketplace
     1. Industry Controls
     2. Consumer Awareness
   C. Food Safety in the Kitchen
     1. Safe Handling of Meats and Poultry
     2. Safe Handling of Seafood
     3. Other Precautions and Procedures
   D. Food Safety While Traveling
   E. Advances in Food Safety
     1. Irradiation
     2. Consumer Concerns about Irradiation
     3. Regulation of Irradiation
     4. Other Pasteurizing Systems
II. Nutritional Adequacy of Foods and Diets
   A. Obtaining Nutrient Information
   B. Minimizing Nutrient Losses
III. Environmental Contaminants
   A. Harmfulness of Environmental Contaminants
     1. Methylmercury
     2. PBB and PCB
   B. Guidelines for Consumers
IV. Natural Toxicants in Foods
V. Pesticides
   A. Hazards and Regulation of Pesticides
     1. Hazards of Pesticides
     2. Regulation of Pesticides
     3. Pesticides from Other Countries
   B. Monitoring Pesticides
     1. Food in the Fields
     2. Food on the Plate
   C. Consumer Concerns
     1. Minimizing Risks
     2. Alternatives to Pesticides
     3. Organically Grown Crops
VI. Food Additives
   A. Regulations Governing Additives
     1. The GRAS List
     2. The Delaney Clause
     3. Margin of Safety
     4. Risks versus Benefits
   B. Intentional Food Additives
     1. Antimicrobials
     2. Antioxidants
     3. Colors
     4. Flavors
     5. Sugar Alternatives
     6. Texture and Stability
     7. Nutrients
   C. Indirect Food Additives
     1. Acrylamide
     2. Food Packaging
     3. Dioxins
     4. Decaffeinated Coffee
     5. Hormones
     6. Antibiotics
VII. Consumer Concerns about Water
   A. Sources of Drinking Water
   B. Water Systems and Regulations
     1. Home Water Treatments
     2. Bottled Water
VIII. Food Biotechnology
   A. The Promises of Genetic Engineering
     1. Extended Shelf Life
     2. Improved Nutrient Composition
     3. Efficient Food Processing
     4. Efficient Drug Delivery
     5. Genetically Assisted Agriculture
     6. Other Possibilities
   B. The Potential Problems and Concerns
   C. FDA Regulations

Summing Up

Millions of people suffer mild to life-threatening symptoms caused by 1._____ illnesses. Most of these illnesses can be prevented by storing and cooking foods at their proper 2._____ and by preparing them in 3._____ conditions. Irradiation of certain foods protects consumers from foodborne illnesses, but it also raises some 4._____.

In the marketplace, 5._____ _____, the *Dietary Guidelines for Americans*, and MyPlate all help consumers learn about nutrition and how to plan healthy diets. At home, consumers can minimize nutrient losses from fruits and vegetables by refrigerating them, washing them before 6._____ them, storing them in

airtight containers, and cooking them for short times in 7._____ water.

    Foods may become contaminated as 8._____ enter the air, land, and sea. So far, the hazards

appear relatively 9._____. In all cases, two principles apply. First, remain alert to the possibility of

contamination of foods, and keep an ear open for public health 10._____ and advice.

Second, eat a 11._____ of foods. Varying food choices is an effective defensive strategy against the

12._____ of toxins in the body. Each food eaten 13.*dilutes* contaminants that may be

present in other components of the diet.

    Natural toxicants include the 14._____ in cabbage, cyanogens in lima beans, and solanine in

potatoes. These examples of naturally occurring toxicants illustrate two familiar principles. First, any substance can

be 15._____ when consumed in excess. Second, poisons are poisons, whether made by people or by

16._____. Remember, it is not the source of a chemical that makes it hazardous, but its chemical

17._____ and the quantity consumed.

    Pesticides can safely improve crop yields when used according to 18._____, but they can

also be hazardous when used inappropriately. The FDA tests both domestic and imported foods for pesticide

19._____ in the fields and in market basket surveys of foods prepared table ready. Alternative farming

methods may allow farmers to grow crops with few or no 20._____.

    On the whole, the benefits of food additives seem to justify the 21._____ associated with their use. The

22._____ regulates the use of the intentional additives. Incidental additives sometimes get into foods during

processing, but rarely present a 23._____, although some processes such as treating livestock with

hormones and 24._____ raise consumer concerns.

    Like foods, 25._____ may contain infectious microorganisms, environmental contaminants, pesticide

residues, and additives. The 26._____ monitors the safety of the public water system, but many consumers choose

home water-treatment systems or 27._____ water instead of tap water.

Chapter Study Questions

1. To what extent does food poisoning present a real hazard to consumers eating U.S. foods? How often does it occur?

2. Distinguish between the two types of foodborne illnesses and provide an example of each. Describe several measures that help prevent foodborne illnesses.

3. What special precautions apply to meats? To seafood?

4. How can people minimize nutrient losses in the kitchen?

5. What is meant by a "persistent" contaminant of foods? Describe how contaminants get into foods and build up in the food chain.

6. What dangers do natural toxicants present?

7. How do pesticides become a hazard to the food supply, and how are they monitored? In what ways can people reduce the concentrations of pesticides in and on foods that they prepare?

8. What is the difference between a GRAS substance and a recently approved food additive? Give examples of each. Name and describe the different classes of additives.

Key Terms Practice

To complete the crossword puzzle, identify the key term that best matches each definition.

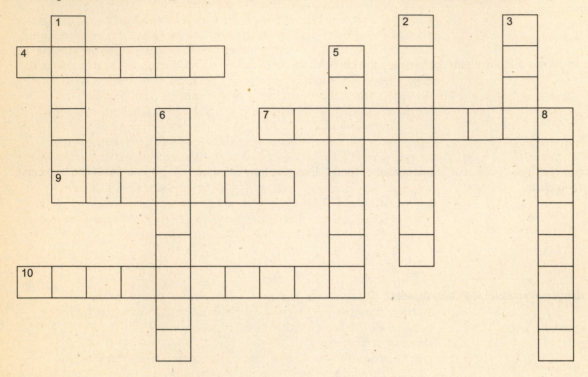

Across:

4. The condition of being free from harm or danger.
7. Two or more cases of a similar illness resulting from the ingestion of a common food.
9. A class of chemical pollutants created as by-products of chemical manufacturing, incineration, chlorine bleaching of paper pulp, and other industrial processes.
10. A substance that causes cancer.

Down:

1. A source of danger; used to refer to circumstances in which harm is possible under normal conditions of use.
2. Salts added to food to prevent botulism often used to preserve meats.
3. A measure of the probability and severity of harm.
5. A microorganism capable of producing disease.
6. The ability of a substance to harm living organisms.
8. Salts containing sulfur that are added to foods to prevent spoilage.

227

Match the key terms with their definitions.

11. _____ additives

12. _____ bioaccumulation

13. _____ contaminants

14. _____ cross-contamination

15. _____ foodborne illnesses

16. _____ irradiation

17. _____ preservatives

18. _____ residues

19. _____ solanine

20. _____ ultrahigh temperature treatment

a. illnesses transmitted to human beings through food and water, caused by either an infectious agent or a poisonous substance

b. sterilizing a food by brief exposure to temperatures above those normally used

c. the contamination of food by bacteria that occurs when the food comes into contact with surfaces previously touched by raw meat, poultry, or seafood

d. sterilizing a food by exposure to energy waves, similar to ultraviolet light and microwaves; sometimes called ionizing radiation

e. substances that make a food impure and unsuitable for ingestion

f. the accumulation of contaminants in the flesh of animals high on the food chain

g. a poisonous narcotic-like substance present in potato peels and sprouts

h. whatever remains; in the case of pesticides, those amounts that remain on or in foods when people buy and use them

i. substances not normally consumed as foods but added to food either intentionally or by accident

j. antimicrobial agents, antioxidants, and other additives that retard spoilage or maintain desired qualities, such as softness in baked goods

21. _____ Acceptable Daily Intake

22. _____ bacteriophages

23. _____ bovine growth hormone

24. _____ genotoxicant

25. _____ GRAS

26. _____ incidental additives

27. _____ intentional food additives

28. _____ nitrosamines

29. _____ organic halogens

30. _____ potable

a. additives intentionally added to foods, such as nutrients, colors, and preservatives

b. food additives that have long been in use and are believed to be safe

c. derivatives of nitrites that may be formed in the stomach when nitrites combine with amines; they are carcinogenic in animals

d. viruses that infect bacteria

e. organic compounds containing one or more atoms of fluorine, chlorine, iodine, or bromine

f. substances that can get into food as a result of contact during growing, processing, packaging, storing, cooking, or some other stage before the foods are consumed

g. a substance that mutates or damages genetic material

h. a hormone produced naturally in the pituitary gland of a cow that promotes growth and milk production; now produced for agricultural use by bacteria

i. suitable for drinking

j. the estimated amount of a sweetener that individuals can safely consume each day over the course of a lifetime without adverse effect

Sample Test Questions

Select the best answer for each question.

1. A term used to describe circumstances in which danger is possible under normal conditions of use is:
   a. *pesticide.*
   b. *risk.*
   c. *hazard.*
   d. *toxicity.*

2. The ability of a substance to harm living organisms is called:
   a. toxicity.
   b. a hazard.
   c. risk.
   d. irradiation.

3. A measure of the probability and severity of harm is called:
   a. toxicity.
   b. hazardousness.
   c. un-safety.
   d. risk.

4. Consumers rely on monitoring agencies to set _____ standards.
   a. risk
   b. hazard
   c. safety
   d. benefit

5. First on the FDA's list of priority concerns related to food is:
   a. foodborne infection.
   b. environmental contaminants.
   c. pesticide residues.
   d. food additives.
   e. food toxicants.

6. Foodborne illnesses are:
   a. minor irritations.
   b. transmitted from one human being to another.
   c. caused by an infectious agent or a poisonous substance.
   d. a and b
   e. b and c

7. Microorganisms capable of causing disease are called:
   a. intoxicants.
   b. pathogens.
   c. residues.
   d. additives.

8. Possible symptoms of foodborne illness that require medical help include:
   a. bloody diarrhea.
   b. diarrhea lasting more than 3 days.
   c. difficulty breathing or swallowing.
   d. fever lasting more than 24 hours.
   e. All of the above

9. Common foodborne pathogens include:
   a. *Salmonella*.
   b. *Campylobacter jejuni*.
   c. solanine.
   d. a and b
   e. a, b and c

10. The most common food toxin is produced by:
    a. *Staphylococcus aureus*.
    b. *Clostridium botulinum*.
    c. *Listeria*.
    d. *Escherichia coli*.

11. Pasteurization is a heat process that:
    a. sterilizes food.
    b. causes exposure to energy waves.
    c. kills bacteria that cause spoilage.
    d. inactivates some microorganisms in food.

12. Which of the following statements is true regarding Hazard Analysis Critical Control Points (HACCP)?
    a. It is a plan to control food pesticide use.
    b. It requires food manufacturers to implement controls to prevent foodborne disease.
    c. It is a plan designed to eliminate all use of ultrahigh temperature treatment.
    d. It is used to provide guidance on food safety in the home kitchen to consumers.

13. When cooked foods come in contact with surfaces touched by raw meat, this is called:
    a. pasteurization.
    b. cross-contamination.
    c. irradiation.
    d. bioaccumulation.

14. To avoid foodborne illnesses at home:
    a. keep a clean, safe kitchen.
    b. avoid cross-contamination.
    c. keep hot foods hot.
    d. keep cold foods cold.
    e. All of the above

15. Which of the following should you do to avoid cross-contamination?
    a. Wash raw meat and poultry.
    b. Rinse cutting boards after cutting raw meat.
    c. Do not wash fruits and vegetables.
    d. Separate raw, cooked, and ready-to-eat foods.

16. Which food item is the **least** likely to present a foodborne illness risk?
    a. Fresh orange
    b. Pasteurized cookie dough
    c. Chopped salad mixture
    d. Ground turkey burger

17. Which of the following statements is true?
    a. All types of food pathogens are detected by odor.
    b. All sushi is dangerous to eat.
    c. Freezing fish can kill all worms and worm eggs.
    d. Eating raw oysters can be dangerous.

18. Foods that are frequently unsafe include:
    a. peeled fruit, high-sugar foods, and steaming-hot foods.
    b. soft cheeses, salad bar items, and hamburgers.
    c. raw milk, raw sprouts, and undercooked eggs.
    d. sandwiches, unwashed berries, and grapes.

19. Nausea, vomiting, and other intestinal problems caused by consuming contaminated food or water are called:
    a. travelers' diarrhea.
    b. indigestion.
    c. dysentery.
    d. gas.

20. What treatment controls mold in grains, sterilizes spices and teas, and controls insects in fresh fruits and vegetables?
    a. Irradiation
    b. Pasteurization
    c. Ultrahigh temperature treatment
    d. Microwaving

21. The major source of heavy metal contaminants in the food chain is:
    a. industry.
    b. agriculture.
    c. nature.
    d. microorganisms.

22. What organization regulates the presence of contaminants in foods?
    a. USPS
    b. FAO
    c. EPA
    d. FDA

23. Chemicals used to control insects, weeds, and fungi on plants are:
    a. additives.
    b. pesticides.
    c. organic halogens.
    d. residues.

24. A poisonous, narcotic-like substance present in potato peels and sprouts is called:
    a. an organic halogen.
    b. solanine.
    c. polybrominated biphenyl.
    d. a cyanogen.

25. Food additives are the concern of the:
    a. GRAS.
    b. USDA.
    c. FDA.
    d. CFC.

26. Substances widely used for many years without apparent ill effects are on the _____ list.
    a. FDA
    b. GRAS
    c. Delaney
    d. Additive Safety

230

27. The Delaney Clause states that no additives known to cause cancer in:
    a. animals or people at any dose level can be used.
    b. people at any dose level can be used.
    c. animals or people at one-gram levels can be used.
    d. people at one-gram levels can be used.

28. Food additives may be used to:
    a. disguise faulty products.
    b. deceive customers.
    c. destroy nutrients.
    d. enhance flavor.

29. Antimicrobial agents protect foods against:
    a. oxidation.
    b. organisms.
    c. radiation.
    d. pesticides.

30. Indirect additives typically find their way into food as a result of:
    a. enrichment/fortification requirements.
    b. home cooking errors.
    c. manufacturing procedures.
    d. advertising gimmicks.

31. An **un**safe way to thaw meats and poultry is:
    a. at room temperature.
    b. in cool water.
    c. in the refrigerator.
    d. in the microwave.

Short Answer Questions

1. Symptoms of foodborne illness that is serious enough to require medical care include:

    a.

    b.

    c.

    d.

    e.

    f.

    g.

    h.

    i.

2. Four actions that consumers can take to help prevent foodborne illnesses when dining out are:

    a.

    b.

    c.

    d.

3. Four simple steps that can prevent foodborne illness are:

    a.   c.

    b.   d.

4. Four ways that the use of low-dose irradiation protects consumers from foodborne illnesses are:

   a.

   b.

   c.

   d.

5. Four ways that consumers can minimize nutrient losses from fruits and vegetables are by:

   a.

   b.

   c.

   d.

6. Four fish that are relatively high in mercury are:

   a.   c.

   b.   d.

7. Seven seafood choices that are relatively low in mercury are:

   a.   e.

   b.   f.

   c.   g.

   d.

8. Nine fish that are relatively high in omega-3 fatty acids and low in mercury are:

   a.   f.

   b.   g.

   c.   h.

   d.   i.

   e.

9. Three natural toxicants and their food sources are:

   a.   c.

   b.

10. Two organizations that regulate the use of pesticides are:

    a.   b.

11. To receive permission to use a new additive, a manufacturer must satisfy the FDA in three ways by demonstrating that the additive is:

    a.   c.

    b.

12. The FDA prohibits the use of food additives when:

   a.

   b.

   c.

   d.

13. Four appropriate uses of nutrient additives are to:

   a.

   b.

   c.

   d.

14. Two sources of drinking water are:

   a.   b.

15. The _____ regulates the safety of public water; the _____ regulated bottled water.

◌ **Chapter 19 Answer Key** ◌

Summing Up

1. foodborne
2. temperatures
3. sanitary
4. concerns
5. food labels
6. cutting
7. minimal
8. pollutants
9. small
10. announcements
11. variety
12. accumulation
13. dilutes
14. goitrogens
15. toxic
16. nature
17. structure
18. regulations
19. residues
20. pesticides
21. risks
22. FDA
23. hazard
24. antibiotics
25. water
26. EPA
27. bottled

Chapter Study Questions

1. Foodborne illness is the leading food safety concern. An estimated 48 million people per year experience foodborne illness. More than 100,000 of them are hospitalized, and for 3,000 of them it is fatal.

2. Two types of foodborne illnesses are those caused by an infectious agent (foodborne infection)—for example, *Campylobacter jejuni*; and those caused by a poisonous substance (food intoxication)—for example, the toxin produced by *Clostridium botulinum*. Measures to prevent them include keeping hands, surfaces, and utensils clean when handling food; separating raw meats, poultry, eggs, and seafood from other foods to avoid cross-contamination; cooking foods thoroughly (using appropriate temperatures and times) to kill microbes, and then keeping hot foods hot enough to prevent their growth; and refrigerating foods promptly and keeping cold foods cold enough to retard microbial growth.

3. Wash all surfaces that have been in contact with raw meats, poultry, eggs, fish, and shellfish before reusing; serve cooked meats, poultry, and seafood on a clean plate. Separate raw meats and seafood from those that have been cooked. Do not consume uncooked marinade that was in contact with raw meat. When cooking meats, use a thermometer to test the internal temperature, and cook to the temperature indicated for that particular meat. Cook hamburgers to at least medium well-done. Cook stuffing separately or stuff poultry just prior to cooking. Do not cook large cuts of meat or turkey in a microwave oven. Cook seafood thoroughly. When serving meats and seafood, maintain temperature of 140 degrees or higher, and heat leftovers thoroughly to least 165 degrees.

4. Refrigerate fruits and vegetables; wash them before cutting them; prepare vegetables by steaming, microwaving, or including them in soups or casseroles that incorporate the cooking water; store them in airtight containers and cook for short periods of time in minimum water.

5. Stubborn or enduring continuance; the quality of persisting, rather than breaking down, in the bodies of animals and human beings. Contaminants get into foods when heavy metals and other contaminants released through industrial processes into the soil, air, and water are absorbed by plants. People either eat the plants (e.g., fruits and vegetables) or animals that have eaten the plants. Toxins in the food chain accumulate: a person whose principal animal-protein source is fish may consume about 100 pounds of fish in a year, and these fish will have consumed a few tons of plant-eating fish in the course of their lifetimes; the plant eaters will have consumed several tons of photosynthetic producer organisms. If the producer organisms have become contaminated with toxic chemicals, these chemicals become more concentrated in the bodies of the fish that consume them. If none of the chemicals are lost along the way, one person ultimately eats the same amount of contaminant as was present in the original several tons of producer organisms.

6. Poisonous mushrooms are natural yet can be dangerous when eaten. Cabbage, turnips, mustard greens, and radishes contain small quantities of goitrogens that can enlarge the thyroid gland; this can cause problems if a person with a thyroid problem consumes large quantities of these foods. Lima beans and some fruit seeds contain cyanogens that, if activated, can produce the deadly poison cyanide. Potatoes contain small amounts of natural poisons such as solanine. Poisons are poisons whether made by man or by nature.

7. Pesticides may become hazardous by remaining on crops, polluting water, contaminating the soil, and accumulating in the tissues of animals. The EPA determines what levels of pesticide residues in the food supply

are considered acceptable. The FDA is responsible for enforcing adherence to this tolerance level, and monitors pesticide residues by collecting samples of foods and testing crops taken directly from the fields. The FDA also monitors pesticide intakes by consumers through its Total Diet Study, in which common foods are purchased from grocery stores, prepared, and then tested for pesticides and other contaminants. To reduce pesticides: Purchase a variety of produce without holes, and possibly choose organic versions of the items most likely to have residues. Remove/discard fat from meat, skin from poultry and fish, pan drippings, and outer leaves of leafy vegetables. Wash and rinse fresh produce thoroughly, removing peels from waxed items or those most likely to be contaminated.

8. A GRAS substance (such as salt) is accepted as safe based on long experience consistent with the belief that it is not hazardous, whereas a new food additive (such as bacteriophage preparations) has been chemically tested to ensure its effectiveness and safety. Types of food additives include antimicrobial agents, which prevent growth of microorganisms; antioxidants, which delay/prevent oxidative damage (e.g. rancidity); colors and flavors, which enhance appearance and taste, respectively; emulsifiers and gums, which improve consistency by thickening or stabilizing the food; and nutrients (vitamins and minerals).

Key Terms Practice

1. hazard	9. dioxins	17. j	25. b
2. nitrites	10. carcinogen	18. h	26. f
3. risk	11. i	19. g	27. a
4. safety	12. f	20. b	28. c
5. pathogen	13. e	21. j	29. e
6. toxicity	14. c	22. d	30. i
7. outbreaks	15. a	23. h	
8. sulfites	16. d	24. g	

Sample Test Questions

1. c (p. 623)	9. d (p. 625)	17. d (p. 631)	25. c (p. 642)
2. a (p. 623)	10. a (p. 626)	18. c (p. 632)	26. b (p. 642)
3. d (p. 623)	11. d (p. 626)	19. a (p. 632)	27. a (p. 642)
4. c (p. 624)	12. b (p. 626)	20. a (p. 632)	28. d (p. 642-643)
5. a (p. 624)	13. b (p. 628)	21. a (pp. 634, 635)	29. b (p. 643-644)
6. c (p. 625)	14. e (pp. 627-628)	22. d (p. 636)	30. c (p. 646)
7. b (p. 626)	15. d (p. 628)	23. b (p. 637)	31. a (p. 629)
8. e (p. 625)	16. a (p. 629)	24. b (p. 637)	

Short Answer Questions

1. bloody diarrhea; diarrhea lasting more than 3 days; difficulty breathing; difficulty swallowing; double vision; fever lasting more than 24 hours; headache, muscle stiffness, and fever; numbness, muscle weakness, and tingling sensations in the skin; rapid heart rate, fainting, and dizziness

2. wash hands with hot, soapy water before meals; expect clean tabletops, dinnerware, utensils, and food preparation areas; expect cooked foods to be served piping hot and salads to be fresh and cold; refrigerate take-home items within 2 hours and use leftovers within 3-4 days

3. clean, separate, cook, chill

4. controlling mold in grains; sterilizing spices and teas for storage at room temperature; controlling insects and extending shelf life in fresh fruits and vegetables; destroying harmful bacteria in fresh and frozen beef, poultry, lamb, and pork

5. refrigerating them, washing them before cutting them, storing them in airtight containers, cooking them for short times in minimal water

6. tilefish, swordfish, king mackerel, shark

7. cod, haddock, pollock, salmon, sole, tilapia, most shellfish

8. anchovies, herring, lake trout, mackerel, pollock, salmon, sardines, smelt, tilapia

9. goitrogens (cabbage, bok choy, turnips, mustard greens, kale, brussels sprouts, cauliflower, broccoli, kohlrabi, radishes); cyanogens (lima beans, fruit seeds); solanine (potatoes)

10. EPA, FDA

11. effective, detectable and measurable in the final food product, safe

12. they are used to disguise faulty or inferior products; they are used to deceive the consumer; use would significantly destroy nutrients; effects can be achieved by economical, sound manufacturing processes instead

13. correct dietary deficiencies known to result in diseases; restore nutrients to levels found in the food before storage, handling, and processing; balance the vitamin, mineral, and protein contents of a food in proportion to the energy content; correct nutritional inferiority in a food that replaces a more nutritious traditional food

14. surface water, groundwater

15. EPA, FDA

ʚ Chapter 20 – Hunger and the Global Environment ɞ

Chapter Outline

I. Hunger in the United States
  A. Defining Hunger in the United States
    1. Food Poverty
    2. Obesity Paradox
  B. Relieving Hunger in the United States
    1. Federal Food Assistance Programs
    2. National Food Recovery Programs
    3. Community Efforts
II. World Hunger
  A. Food Shortages
    1. Political Turbulence
    2. Armed Conflicts
    3. Natural Disasters
  B. Poverty and Overpopulation
    1. Population Growth Leads to Hunger and Poverty
    2. Hunger and Poverty Lead to Population Growth
    3. Breaking the Cycle
III. Malnutrition
  A. Nutrient Deficiencies
  B. Growth Failure
    1. Wasting of Kwashiorkor
    2. Stunting of Marasmus
  C. Rehabilitation
IV. The Global Environment
  A. Hunger and Environment Connections
    1. Planting Crops
    2. Raising Livestock
    3. Fishing
    4. Energy Overuse
    5. Water Misuse
    6. Biodiversity
    7. Food Waste
  B. Sustainable Solutions
    1. Sustainable Agriculture
    2. Sustainable Development
    3. Sustainable Actions
V. Environmentally Friendly Food Choices
  A. Choice: Animal or Vegetable?
  B. Choice: Global or Local?
    1. Defining *Local*
    2. Eco-Friendly Miles
  C. Other Food-Related Choices

Summing Up

Food insecurity and hunger are widespread in the United States among those living in 1._____. Ironically, hunger and poverty coexist with 2._____. Government assistance programs help to 3._____ poverty and hunger. Food 4._____ programs and other community efforts also provide some relief.

Natural causes such as drought, flood, and pests and political causes such as 5._____ _____ and government policies all contribute to the extreme hunger and poverty seen in the developing countries. In addition, 6._____ means more mouths to feed, which worsens the problems of poverty and 7._____. Poverty and hunger, in turn, encourage parents to have more 8._____ to help support the family. Breaking this cycle requires improving the 9._____ status of the people and providing them with health care, 10._____, and family planning.

Hunger leads to 11._____, which appears most evident in nutrient deficiencies and 12._____ failure. Children suffering from 13._____ _____ (recent severe food deprivation) may be underweight for their height, while those experiencing 14._____ _____ (long-term food deprivation) are short for their age. Problems resulting from nutrient deficiencies include preterm births and low birth weights (15._____), stillbirths and 16._____ (iodine), blindness (17._____), and growth failure (18._____). Treatment should be individualized to ensure rapid 19._____ _____ and correct nutrient deficiencies.

Environmental 20._____ reduces our ability to produce enough food to feed the world's people. The rapid increase in the world's 21._____ exacerbates the situation. The global 22._____, which supports all life, is deteriorating, largely because of our irresponsible use of resources and 23._____. Governments, businesses, and all individuals have many opportunities to make environmentally conscious 24._____, which may help solve the hunger problem, improve the quality of life, and generate jobs. Personal choices, made by many people, can have a great 25._____.

Chapter Study Questions

1. Identify some reasons why hunger is present in a country as wealthy as the United States.

2. Identify some reasons why hunger is present in the developing countries of the world.

3. Describe the consequences of nutrient and energy inadequacies.

4. Are the conventional methods used to grow food crops environmentally friendly? Why or why not?

5. Discuss the different paths by which rich and poor countries can attack the problems of world hunger and the environment.

6. Describe some strategies that consumers can use to minimize negative environmental impacts when shopping for food and preparing meals.

238

Key Terms Practice

To complete the crossword puzzle, identify the key term that best matches each definition.

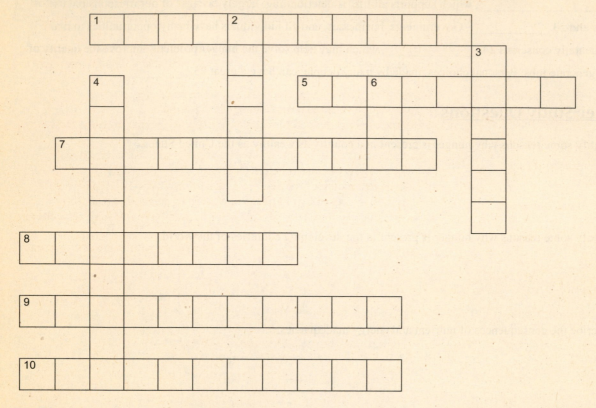

Across:
1. Severe malnutrition characterized by failure to grow and develop, edema, changes in the pigmentation of hair and skin, fatty liver, anemia, and apathy.
5. A facility that collects and distributes food donations to authorized organizations feeding the hungry.
7. Neighborhoods and communities characterized by limited access to nutritious and affordable foods.
8. Severe malnutrition characterized by poor growth, dramatic weight loss, loss of body fat and muscle, and apathy.
9. Able to continue indefinitely; using resources at such a rate that the Earth can keep on replacing them and producing pollutants at a rate with which the environment and human cleanup efforts can keep pace, so that no net accumulation of pollution occurs.
10. Coal, oil, and natural gas.

Down:
2. Consequence of food insecurity that, because of prolonged, involuntary lack of food, results in discomfort, illness, weakness, or pain that goes beyond the usual uneasy sensation.
3. Widespread and extreme scarcity of food in an area that causes starvation and death in a large portion of the population.
4. A sharp rise in the rates of hunger and malnutrition, usually set off by a shock to either the supply of, or demand for, food and a sudden spike in food prices.
6. The administration of a simple solution of sugar, salt, and water, taken by mouth, to treat dehydration caused by diarrhea.

Match the key terms with their definitions.

11. _____ acute malnutrition

12. _____ chronic malnutrition

13. _____ emergency shelters

14. _____ food insecurity

15. _____ food insufficiency

16. _____ food poverty

17. _____ food recovery

18. _____ nonpoint water pollution

19. _____ soup kitchens

20. _____ sustainable agriculture

a. limited or uncertain access to foods of sufficient quality or quantity to sustain a healthy and active life

b. malnutrition caused by long-term food deprivation; characterized in children by short height for age (stunting)

c. hunger resulting from inadequate access to available food for various reasons, including inadequate resources, political obstacles, social disruptions, poor weather conditions, and lack of transportation

d. programs that provide prepared meals to be eaten on site

e. facilities that are used to provide temporary housing

f. collecting wholesome food for distribution to low-income people who are hungry

g. malnutrition caused by recent severe food restriction; characterized in children by underweight for height (wasting)

h. an inadequate amount of food due to a lack of resources

i. water pollution caused by runoff from all over an area rather than from discrete "point" sources (e.g., the pollution caused by runoff from agricultural fields)

j. ability to produce food indefinitely, with little or no harm to the environment

Sample Test Questions

Select the best answer for each question.

1. An estimated 1 out of every _____ people worldwide experiences persistent hunger.
   a. 4
   b. 6
   c. 8
   d. 10
   e. 20

2. Certain access to enough food for people to sustain a healthy and active life at all times is:
   a. food recovery.
   b. food security.
   c. food management.
   d. food access.

3. Which of the following statements is true regarding food availability?
   a. Due to agricultural bounty in the U.S., hunger is not a problem.
   b. Due to enormous wealth in the U.S., food insecurity is not an issue.
   c. An estimated 15% of people in the U.S. live in poverty and cannot afford to buy enough food.
   d. One out of 30 households in the U.S. experiences hunger or the threat of hunger.

4. The limited or uncertain access to foods of sufficient quality or quantity to sustain a healthy life is:
   a. food poverty.
   b. hunger.
   c. food recovery.
   d. food insecurity.

5. People who have too little food and try to stretch their limited resources by eating small meals or skipping meals are experiencing:
   a. high food security.
   b. food insufficiency.
   c. food assistance.
   d. famine.

6. Reasons for food poverty include:
   a. illnesses and disabilities.
   b. unemployment, low-paying jobs, and medical expenses.
   c. abuse of alcohol and other drugs.
   d. a and b
   e. a, b and c

7. Which of the following statements is true about hunger?
   a. People who are hungry are underweight.
   b. The highest rates of obesity occur among those living in the greatest poverty.
   c. People who are obese have plenty of income to purchase large amounts of food.
   d. Food insecure people who do not participate in food assistance programs have lower rates of obesity.

8. The largest federal food assistance program is:
   a. WIC.
   b. the School Lunch Program.
   c. Meals on Wheels.
   d. the Supplemental Nutrition Assistance Program.

9. Collecting wholesome food for distribution to low-income people who are hungry is:
   a. food recovery.
   b. food security.
   c. food banking.
   d. food pantries.

10. Common methods of food recovery include:
    a. field gleaning and perishable food rescue.
    b. prepared food rescue and nonperishable food collection.
    c. dumpster food rescue and soup kitchens.
    d. a and b
    e. a, b and c

11. Collecting crops from fields that have already been harvested is specifically called:
    a. food insecurity.
    b. field gleaning.
    c. food rescue.
    d. food collection.

12. Extreme scarcity of food that causes starvation is:
    a. extinction.
    b. deforestation.
    c. sustainable.
    d. famine.
    e. poverty.

13. To help achieve rapid weight gain, _____ are distributed to children worldwide.
    a. large containers of rice
    b. bottles of clean water
    c. vitamin A supplements
    d. ready-to-use therapeutic food packets

14. Administration of a sugar, salt, and water solution is called:
    a. ORT.
    b. FDA.
    c. WHO.
    d. RUTF.

15. The primary cause of hunger is:
    a. lack of education about food selection and preparation.
    b. abuse of alcohol and other drugs.
    c. depression.
    d. poverty.
    e. mental illness.

16. Which of the following is an example of a sustainable agricultural practice?
    a. Increasing the quantity of fertilizer applied to the soil
    b. Irrigating all fields regularly
    c. Plowing in the same direction on all fields
    d. Feeding livestock on the open range

17. A sharp rise in rates of hunger and malnutrition is:
    a. known as a food crisis.
    b. usually initiated by a drop in food prices.
    c. unlikely to occur at the present time.
    d. called a famine.

18. Which of the following statements is true regarding poverty and overpopulation?
    a. Women living in poverty have fewer children than women with financial means.
    b. Women in poverty are treated well by men.
    c. In some areas, children raised in poverty are economic assets.
    d. Families living in poverty choose to live the way they do.

19. Which statement is true?
    a. The U.S. food industry consumes about 8% of the total energy used by the nation.
    b. The EPA estimates that current farming practices cause 70% of the pollution in U.S. rivers and streams.
    c. In the U.S., more cropland is used to produce grains for people than for livestock to eat.
    d. Though currently wild-caught fish quantities are keeping pace with consumption, this may change.

20. Using resources at a rate at which the earth can continue replacing them is called:
    a. degradation.
    b. sustainable use.
    c. population growth.
    d. carrying capacity.

21. Urgent needs for all nations' economies include:
    a. hunger relief and population stabilization.
    b. environmental preservation and sustainable resources.
    c. nutrition education and food giveaways.
    d. a and b
    e. a, b and c

22. Which segments of society can have an impact in fighting hunger, poverty, and environmental degradation?
    a. Federal and state governments
    b. Companies and educators
    c. Individuals
    d. a and b
    e. a, b and c

23. Fossil fuels include:
    a. ozone.
    b. coal.
    c. oil.
    d. a and b
    e. b and c

24. If a person responds positively to the question, "Our children are not eating enough because we couldn't afford food," this indicates:
    a. food withholding.
    b. food insecurity.
    c. poor parenting.
    d. food security.

25. Diseases of poverty in malnourished children include:
    a. parasitic diseases.
    b. measles.
    c. acute respiratory illnesses.
    d. malaria.
    e. all of the above

26. Severe malnutrition characterized by failure to grow and develop, edema, and pigmentation changes is:
    a. chronic malnutrition.
    b. kwashiorkor.
    c. marasmus.
    d. cretinism.

27. The severe deprivation of food over a long time that causes stunting is:
    a. acute malnutrition.
    b. kwashiorkor.
    c. bulimia.
    d. marasmus.

28. Water pollution caused by runoff from all over an area rather than from a specific source is:
    a. nonpoint water pollution.
    b. relatively easy to control.
    c. industrial water pollution.
    d. not a significant source of water pollution.

242

29. Intense demands placed on water resources by human activities are collectively known as:
    a. water stress.
    b. water misuse.
    c. biodiversity.
    d. water abuse.

30. Food waste:
    a. has a minor environmental impact.
    b. produces methane and carbon dioxide.
    c. is minimal due to worldwide hunger.
    d. enhances sustainability.
    e. All of the above

Short Answer Questions

1. Two food security categories are their definitions are:

   a.

   b.

2. Two food insecurity categories and their definitions are:

   a.

   b.

3. Four common methods of food recovery and their descriptions are:

   a.

   b.

   c.

   d.

4. Two major non-natural causes of famine are:

   a.   b.

5. The first step to breaking the cycle of poverty and overpopulation is improved _____ status.

6. The 4 nutrients most likely to be deficient in human diets are:

   a.   c.

   b.   d.

7. Six diseases of poverty common in underweight children are:

   a.   d.

   b.   e.

   c.   f.

8. Two forms of malnutrition that result in growth failure in children are:

   a.   b.

9. Three things that can be provided to prevent death from diarrheal disease are:

   a.   c.

   b.

10. Two ways in which hunger interacts with the environment are:

    a.

    b.

11. Suggested changes that might reduce fossil fuel energy use by about 50% include:

    a.

    b.

    c.

    d.

    e.

    f.

12. Two products that result from decomposition of food and contribute to greenhouse gases and climate change are:

    a.   b.

13. Four criticisms of the reliance on foods transported long distances are that it is:

    a.   c.

    b.   d.

⊚ Chapter 20 Answer Key ⊚

Summing Up

1. poverty	8. children	14. chronic malnutrition	20. degradation
2. obesity	9. economic	15. iron	21. population
3. relieve	10. education	16. cretinism	22. environment
4. recovery	11. malnutrition	17. vitamin A	23. energy
5. armed conflicts	12. growth	18. zinc	24. choices
6. overpopulation	13. acute malnutrition	19. weight gain	25. impact
7. hunger			

Chapter Study Questions

1. Hunger is present in the U.S. because of the many political, social, and economic factors related to poverty. The primary cause of hunger in the U.S. and other developed countries is food poverty; i.e., people live in hunger because their income is too low to purchase enough food. For those surviving on low incomes, crises such as illness, injury, unemployment, or unexpected expenses may force a decision to reduce food purchases in order to continue to pay fixed expenses such as rent and utilities.

2. Poverty is the primary cause. A second major cause is famine due to political unrest, armed conflict, or natural disasters. Overpopulation contributes to hunger by increasing the demand for food while reducing the land available for food production as cities and industry encroach on farmland.

3. The consequences of nutrient and energy inadequacy include various forms of malnutrition. The most common micronutrient deficiencies are of iron (>30% of the population have iron-deficiency anemia), iodine (which causes cretinism in infants), vitamin A (a cause of blindness), and zinc (20% of the population are at risk). Inadequate food intake in children results in growth failure that may be categorized as kwashiorkor—acute malnutrition characterized by wasting and edema—or marasmus—chronic malnutrition that causes wasting and stunting. These dire outcomes appear to result from deficiencies of many nutrients, including amino acids, potassium, magnesium, zinc, and phosphorus. Such poor-quality diets result in loss of appetite, diminished growth, and inability to resist infection or respond to environmental stresses.

4. No; current agricultural methods damage the environment. Clearing land for agricultural use destroys native ecosystems; fertilizer and eroded soil runoff pollutes fresh water in rivers and lakes and ultimately the ocean. Similarly, herbicides and pesticides pollute air and water, killing native organisms and promoting the evolution of more resistant pests and weeds. Field irrigation increases the saltiness of soil and depletes water supplies.

5. The poor nations need to provide contraceptive technology and family planning information to their citizens, develop better programs to assist the poor, and slow and reverse the destruction of environmental resources. Rich nations need to reduce wasteful and polluting uses of resources and energy and relieve the debt burdens of poor nations.

6. Shoppers can car pool, use mass transit, walk or bicycle to shop, shop less often—make fewer trips, or take turns shopping for each other. Plan how much to buy to minimize food waste. Choose mostly plant foods, and only small portions of animal foods raised in environmentally responsible ways; shop at farmers' markets or roadside stands. Select foods with no, minimal, reusable, or recyclable packages, and carry purchases home in reusable shopping bags. When preparing foods: use a pressure cooker and microwave or stir-fry foods, use the oven and stove top less often, and do without small electrical appliances. Use nondisposable dishes, utensils, and pans to prepare and serve food, and properly store and eat any leftovers.

Key Terms Practice

1. kwashiorkor
2. hunger
3. famine
4. food crisis
5. food bank
6. ORT
7. food deserts
8. marasmus
9. sustainable
10. fossil fuels
11. g
12. b
13. e
14. a
15. h
16. c
17. f
18. i
19. d
20. j

Sample Test Questions

1. c (p. 659)
2. b (p. 660)
3. c (p. 661)
4. d (p. 660)
5. b (p. 661)
6. e (p. 661)
7. b (p. 661-662)
8. d (p. 662)
9. a (p. 663)
10. d (p. 663)
11. b (p. 663)
12. d (p. 664)
13. d (p. 669)
14. a (p. 669-670)
15. d (p. 664)
16. d (pp. 673, 674)
17. a (p. 670)
18. c (p. 666)
19. b (pp. 671-672)
20. b (p. 673)
21. d (p. 673)
22. e (p. 674)
23. e (p. 671)
24. b (p. 660)
25. e (p. 667)
26. b (p. 668)
27. d (pp. 668-669)
28. a (p. 670)
29. a (p. 672)
30. b (p. 673)

Short Answer Questions

1. a. high food security: no indications of food-access problems or limitations
   b. marginal food security: one or two indications of food-access problems but with little or no change in food intake

2. a. low food security: reduced quality of life with little or no indication of reduced food intake;
   b. very low food security: multiple indications of disrupted eating patterns and reduced food intake

3. a. field gleaning: collecting crops from fields that either have already been harvested or are not profitable to harvest
   b. perishable food rescue or salvage: collecting perishable produce from wholesalers and markets
   c. prepared food rescue: collecting prepared foods from commercial kitchens
   d. nonperishable food collection: collecting processed foods from wholesalers and markets

4. political turbulence, armed conflicts

5. economic

6. iron, iodine, vitamin A, zinc

7. dysentery, cholera, pneumonia, whooping cough, measles, malaria

8. kwashiorkor (acute malnutrition), marasmus (chronic malnutrition)

9. adequate sanitation, safe water, oral rehydration therapy

10. food production to feed billions of people around the world damages the environment; a damaged environment cannot support food production to feed billions of people around the world

11. using small machinery and less fuel, replacing fertilizer with cover crops and manure, tilling to reduce soil erosion, reducing consumption of meat and dairy products, limiting transportation distances, combining efficient practices with renewable systems

12. methane, carbon dioxide

13. energetically costly, socially unjust, economically unwise, biologically risky